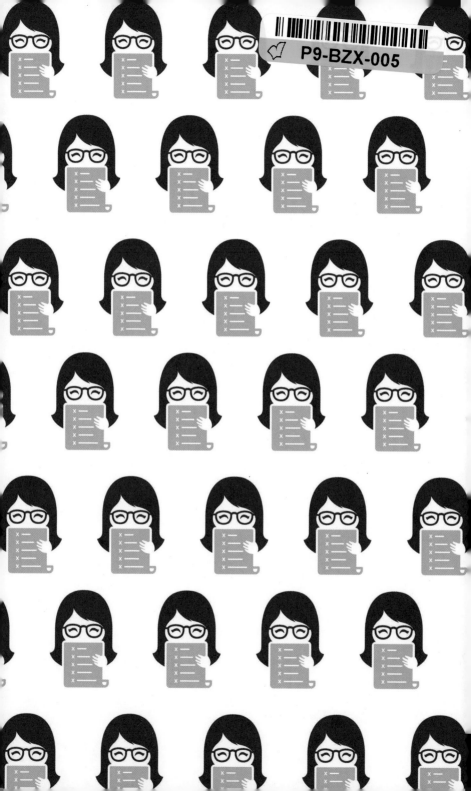

Advance Praise

"Zibby Owens is a genius at throwing a party—the kind where all the guests will like each other, the chatter won't stop, and everybody leaves feeling like they're part of a chic bookish girls club. But with the pandemic throwing a wrench in IRL parties, Zibby found that she was just as at home throwing a party via essay collection and that's what this is: a vertical Rolodex of friends who will remind you that women can, do, and always have had the power to balance entire impossible lives—and still read books. Welcome this explosion of joy onto your bookshelf that is so relevant, so now, and so purely Zibby."

—**LENA DUNHAM**, #1 *New York Times* bestselling author of *Not That Kind of Girl*

"Zibby Owens is a maven and a connector, a book lover whose passion for people and genuine interest in their stories has transformed a global community of readers into an intimate and supportive society of friends. This collection is the product of Zibby's talent, passion, and constant quest to find the stories both big and small that make our lives meaningful. As a mother, as a wife, as a reader, as an author—simply as a human being—I cherished this collection of honest, thought-provoking, and funny essays."

—**ALLISON PATAKI**, *New York Times* bestselling author of *The Queen's Fortune*

"Zibby's essay collection is just like her: warm, inclusive, literary, at times funny, and always refreshingly real. Every piece in here will make you think, shift your perspective, and touch your soul."

—**LORI GOTTLIEB**, *New York Times* bestselling author of *Maybe You Should Talk To Someone: A Therapist, Her Therapist, and Our Lives Revealed*

"Even before COVID-19 changed the way we live and work and communicate with each other, Zibby Owens was already a force for good: promoting books through her 'Moms Don't Have Time to Read Books' podcast and events and bringing people together who shared her passion for reading. Throughout the pandemic, she continued to be The Great Connector, making us all feel less alone during a time of unprecedented anxiety, isolation, and uncertainty. *Moms Don't Have Time To* is the product of the many writers and readers she connected—"virtually"—in lockdown: a network of women encouraging each other, showing up for each other, and supporting each other through both our best and our toughest moments. Funny, moving, and hopeful, these pieces will forever remind us how we all got through this singular moment in history: together, and with a lot of great books!"

—**LAURA ZIGMAN**, bestselling author of *Animal Husbandry* and *Separation Anxiety*

"The perfect reminder for every mom that none of us have it all together, all of us are doing our best and, most important, even your worst days make a great story."

—**NORA McINERNY**, author of *No Happy Endings* and host of popular podcast *Terrible, Thanks for Asking*

"Each of these brilliant essays shines as bright as Zibby Owens herself, who is a Fourth-of-July firework in human form. Actually, I've always wished that everyone could have the opportunity to experience Zibby's pure energy in person. She's a connector of people, a bolt of energy, a burst of unconditional love. But then, after reading this book, I realized you don't actually have to meet Zibby in person to experience her pure Zibbyness. You can read these essays, which she has lovingly nurtured and curated in the midst of both a global pandemic and her own personal losses therein, and feel that Zibby godlight shining through all of our clouded souls."

—**DEBORAH COPAKEN**, *New York Times* bestselling author of *Shutterbabe*, *The Red Book*, and her new upcoming memoir, *Ladyparts*

"This moving collection, curated by Zibby Owens, runs the gamut of human relationships. These essays examine our connection with our bodies, our lovers, our kids, our friends, and our minds. Each one is poignant and sharp, slipping between the mundane and the spiritual, and is utterly refreshing during a time of universal longing and loneliness. *Moms Don't Have Time To* is an absolute gift."

—**STEPHANIE DANLER**, *New York Times* bestselling author of *Sweetbitter* and *Stray*

"Zibby Owens is a force for good in more ways than I can count. In this anthology borne of a longing to connect and heal, she has gathered a group of wise and generous writers—herself included!—who are quite simply the best company. Curl up with this book, and I promise you'll be surrounded by kindred spirits."

—**DANI SHAPIRO**, *New York Times* bestselling author of *Inheritance: A Memoir of Genealogy, Paternity, and Love*

"In a time when we need to feel connected more than ever, Zibby Owens has done what she does best—bring together extraordinary voices in the literary world to give us words that make us feel less alone. This anthology will be one to keep handy for years to come, something to turn to when you just need to be reminded of how perfectly imperfect we all really are."

—**CLAIRE BIDWELL SMITH**, bestselling author of *The Rules of Inheritance* and author of *Anxiety: The Missing Stage of Grief*

"Zibby isn't just a tireless champion for books, she's a community builder who was able to make readers and authors feel less alone during a year of terrible isolation and uncertainty. This collection of warm, relatable, funny, unfailingly honest essays feels like hanging out at a book club full of smart, funny women once the Chardonnay hits. It's the Algonquin Roundtable in yoga pants. As an author and a mom, I'm so glad I found time for *Moms Don't Have Time To*. The dishes, on the other hand . . . "
—**BESS KALB**, bestselling author of *Nobody Will Tell You This But Me*

"From 'Awake, 3:01 a.m.' to 'Sheltering with Ghosts' to 'How to Have Sex with a Germaphobe,' this collection of essays, written in real time during the spring and summer of 2020, is a boon pandemic companion. Writer Zibby Owens has created an anthology full of emotion, humor, and good advice for these troubled times and beyond."
—**LILY KING**, *New York Times* bestselling author of *Writers & Lovers*

"Zibby Owens has assembled some of the best writers around and the result is a hilarious, inspiring collection of essays about all the things we don't have time for, and yet must do to keep ourselves joyful and engaged—or, at the very least, sane. A delightful read from start to finish."
—**J. COURTNEY SULLIVAN**, *New York Times* bestselling author of *Friends and Strangers*

MOMS DON'T HAVE TIME TO

MOMS DON'T HAVE TIME TO

A QUARANTINE ANTHOLOGY

Edited by Zibby Owens

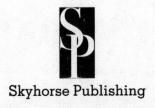

Skyhorse Publishing

Skyhorse Publishing books may be purchased in bulk at special discounts for sales promotion, corporate gifts, fund-raising, or educational purposes. Special editions can also be created to specifications. For details, contact the Special Sales Department, Skyhorse Publishing, 307 West 36th Street, 11th Floor, New York, NY 10018 or info@skyhorsepublishing.com.

Skyhorse® and Skyhorse Publishing® are registered trademarks of Skyhorse Publishing, Inc.®, a Delaware corporation.

Visit our website at www.skyhorsepublishing.com.

10 9 8 7 6 5 4 3 2 1

Library of Congress Cataloging-in-Publication Data is available on file.

Cover design by Jovelyn Valle
Cover photo and art direction by McCain Merren and Nina Vargas

Print ISBN: 978-1-5107-6596-2
Ebook ISBN: 978-1-5107-6597-9

Printed in the United States of America

To my four kids, O, P, S & G, who all requested that they alone get this dedication. (Sorry, guys. You have to share.)

And to Kyle. If it weren't for you, no one would be reading this.

In loving memory of Susan Felice Owens and Marie Felice, Kyle's mother and grandmother, who we lost too soon to COVID-19.

All proceeds of this book will go to the Susan Felice Owens Program for COVID-19 Vaccine Research at Mount Sinai Health System.

TABLE OF CONTENTS

WORK OUT

EAT

HAVE SEX

BREATHE

Author Features

INTRODUCTION

I t shouldn't have been me. I was new to the literary world. Yes, I'd been dancing on its doorstep for decades, freelancing, ghostwriting, opening rejection letters about my novels. But I'd only really gotten immersed in it when I started my literary podcast, *Moms Don't Have Time to Read Books*, two years earlier on a whim. (See the Afterword & Acknowledgments section for the whole story.)

In the midst of the coronavirus pandemic, I found myself pulled to be the hub of author wisdom. It overtook me, this mission to help authors, to connect books to readers, to shine a light on shadowed stories. I felt an enormous responsibility to disseminate information, especially then.

As all the structures of my personal life as a NYC-based, (re)married mother of four slowly circled the drain of the quarantine, my need to serve intensified. I felt like I was in one of those movies about the tsunami in Thailand. I could see the enormous wave coming, yet all I could do was jump up and grab a branch, hoping it would pass beneath me.

The literary community has been my branch.

Before COVID-19 hit, I thought I was busy. I was recording five podcasts a week, mostly in person at home. That meant reading/ skimming five books a week, preparing, researching. (Now, that seems easy.) As the virus neared, I packed up my family, grabbed our important documents, and made plans to leave. Admittedly, I was fortunate to have a place to escape to outside of the city while so many others didn't have that option—and still don't.

As soon as I got the kids, then ages five through twelve, firmly situated in our shelter for the coronavirus, lovies on the pillowcases, devices charged, I got to work. What could I do? I quickly realized that so many authors, like the three hundred plus I'd interviewed intimately, were getting to the finish line of multiyear book-writing journeys only to have their "pub days" and accompanying events pulled. Their paperback releases were canceled. Conferences and speaking engagements, deleted. How would they be able to get the word out?

I sat at the kitchen table as my kids circled about, drawing, fighting, dancing, and eating, and scrolled through all the books coming out. I picked the most intriguing titles and decided to promote them. But that wasn't enough. I woke up at 3:30 a.m. when my six-year-old daughter climbed into bed with us and couldn't fall back asleep. I had to do more. But what?

News reports seeped in. My kids' schools fell like dominoes, one closing, then another, until all four of their schools announced that they'd be closed until the end of April. Little did I know then that many wouldn't even open come fall. This wasn't going to be the two-week exodus I had anticipated or packed for. (Mental note: do not grab "dry clean only" sweaters when packing for a pandemic.) This was going to be for the long haul.

As social distancing morphed into mandated business closures, many people started losing their jobs. GoFundMe campaigns popped up in my inbox for many restaurants and small businesses I cared about. I contributed online like I was playing a carnival game of Whack-a-Mole. As soon as I helped one, another appeared in desperate need. I kept whacking, eventually opening up free sponsorship slots on my podcast to help struggling entities.

I doubled down on helping the literary community in the best way I could: bringing authors to readers. I reached out to the soon-to-be new authors and invited them to be on my new Instagram Live show, *Z-IGTV.* Maybe that would help? I vowed to do five live interviews a day every weekday in ten-minute slots. (*Z-IGTV* has since won media awards.)

Suddenly I was a booker, researcher, producer, and anchor of a morning talk show, all by myself. Plus I still had my podcasts to prepare for. And the kids were waiting for me to play Monopoly. Or paint. Or find that one page of homework that they desperately needed. And could my daughter dye her hair blue? *What?!?*

When a trusted team member suggested I stop doing Instagram Lives since they weren't really boosting my number of followers, I tried to explain that I wasn't doing *any* of it to boost followers or gain more newsletter subscribers, goals from pre-pandemic that I tossed aside as quickly as my high heels. My goal was just to help. Full stop. To give authors a platform. To entertain friends and strangers who were stuck at home, to give them a break from refreshing their horrifying news feeds on their phones, their anxiety spiking. To give away useful things from companies that offered, not to help my business but just to actually give things away and make people happy.

As nurses with bruised faces from N95 masks appeared in the papers and soldiers tromped into my hometown to turn the Jacob Javits Center (where I'd been scheduled to attend BookExpo and to moderate a BookCon event) into a makeshift war hospital, I booked more experts. I skimmed books. I researched authors. I learned. I healed. I joked around "on air" and solicited advice from those far wiser than me. I asked what they were reading.

It still wasn't enough; I kept innovating. My husband, Kyle, and I launched an Instagram Live weekly show called *KZ Time* where we chatted with other literary couples. I started Zibby's Virtual Book Club, which met weekly throughout the summer with half an hour of book club discussion followed by half an hour of author Q&A. (Now it meets every other week.) I recommended books in articles for the

Washington Post, Real Simple, and *Good Morning America.* I went on TV often, many times with Kyle, and passionately explained why I loved certain books.

Finally, I launched *We Found Time,* a magazine for the quarantine. I had been mulling over the idea for months, even before the pandemic hit. Author Claire Gibson and I had sat at my kitchen island and brainstormed how I could take my idea—a magazine with essays about all the things moms didn't have time to do like eat, have sex, work out, breathe, and more—and turn it into something real. We realized it could be entirely written by authors who had been on my podcast. Claire volunteered to help me launch it. Memoirist Elissa Altman, whom I had long admired, joined the team to help edit incoming essays. And then, everything changed.

We pivoted quickly. Instead of launching our online magazine months out as we'd planned guided by the strategic counsel of my friend and consigliere, Maxi Kozler, we rushed it to "press." My old friend, designer Somsara Rielly, gave in to my begging and, working with wunderkind McCain Merren, produced the entire design and launched it in weeks. I took all the pictures for the issues. Nina Vargas, formerly my kids' babysitter and then head of events—which had completely ceased—took care of social media promotion. Jamie Mortimer, my kids' babysitter, my right-hand lady, and a former English major, copy edited. We Found Time?! Yes, we sure did.

My tiny team produced compassionate, timely literary essays. Carolyn Murnick, an author from my podcast, used her years of experience at *New York* magazine and stepped in to help edit and refine the concept. Alice Berman, another author and dear friend, negotiated partnerships. I hosted an online Zoom launch event at which thirty plus authors came to celebrate the release of this new form of entertainment, an antidote to the stress of the changing world.

All the essays we produced during lockdown are in this book. We released them over the course of two months in the most uncertain times we've ever lived through. Everyone juggled their own issues, health concerns, kids, spouses, other work, and more to produce it. I couldn't be more grateful.

It shouldn't have been me at the center of all of this literary action when bestselling authors, career editors, agents, publishers, and journalists would surely have been more qualified. But it was. And I knew I was doing the right thing, even if there wasn't anything quantifiable to show for it. After all, that's not why I was doing any of it.

Sometimes I felt like a medium or a psychic, like I'd been given this precious gift of being a trusted intermediary. I could ignore it and shove it in a closet, or I could place that gift carefully in my hands and showcase it to the world. I trotted it out.

When I saw pictures of overworked doctors in protective bubbles, eerie, empty streets all over the globe, and patients struggling to breathe in overcrowded hospitals, I felt helpless. When readers emailed me to say my *We Found Time* essays were helping, I knew it was all worth it.

I don't have a medical degree. I couldn't stop the pandemic. I couldn't make my life—or anyone else's—go back to normal. I couldn't even explain to my five-year-old son why he couldn't add anything to the Countdown app on my phone because we didn't have any plans to count down to, possibly ever. I couldn't help patients breathe. But I'm glad I could help people at home breathe a little easier, think, connect, smile, and learn. Feel less alone. Feel human.

So that's how *We Found Time* happened, even though my seventy-something-year-old mother told me even *she* didn't have the time to consume all the content I was creating. I wanted the right person to find the right story, quote, or sentence for them.

I may have been stuck inside indefinitely, homeschooling four kids. I may have been overcome with anxiety and fear and sadness and hopelessness at what was befalling our beloved world. I may have been separated from loved ones, family, friends, and community.

I may have been unable to hug, to see, to touch, to smile at others. But I decided to respect that gift—that pull—so others could connect through storytelling. I decided to keep listening to the voice in my head each night that whispered: *how else can I help?*

And I'm so glad I did.

It shouldn't have been me. But it was.

We released the final issue of *We Found Time* on July 27, 2020, when things seemed to be going back to normal and time would be lost again.

That very week COVID-19 struck my family.

My husband Kyle's grandmother, Marie ("Nene") Felice, passed away from COVID-19, which she inadvertently "caught" while hospitalized for a life-threatening heart condition several weeks before. The hospital released her without testing her for COVID-19.

She promptly went home and gave it to her daughter and roommate, my mother-in-law, Susan Owens. At sixty-three, Susan was healthy and newly divorced, a hardworking baker and small business owner who had started a new relationship with a guy with a motorcycle (that she actually dared to ride!). She stopped everything to care for her mother, but quickly caught COVID-19—with a raging fever—herself. When Nene went back into the hospital, now dying from COVID-19, Susan donned a full-body hazmat suit to say goodbye. She stuffed it with ice packs.

The day after her mother passed away, Susan was admitted to the hospital. For the next three weeks she endured horrific health care challenges while fighting COVID-19. A nurse spilled a container of urine on her. No one washed her thick, shining, chest-length, chocolate-brown mane, or even took the time to brush her teeth. COVID-19 tests were jammed up her nostrils daily until her nose grew infected. She lay "prone," upside down, to help open up her lungs, and the nurses forgot about her. This was the one moment, during a phone call, when tears broke through her typical Jersey-girl, "I got this!" fist-pump emoji self.

After three weeks on a cocktail of meds like remdesivir and steroids, her lungs still ended up ravaged. She went on a ventilator and then, when that failed and the doctors in Charlotte ran out of options, she was airlifted to Duke University. She spent another three weeks in the ICU on a ventilator, an ECMO breathing machine, then dialysis for her kidneys, until she had a stroke that ended her valiant fight to live. Kyle, his sister, Stefanie, and I heard the news in our hotel room and began howling as Susan's two well-behaved dogs suddenly attacked each other.

When I first asked Susan if she and Nene wanted to quarantine with us, she had politely demurred. She didn't want to be an imposition, especially with the two dogs, Nya, a black Lab, and Luna, a Husky/Bull Terrier mix who Kyle had rescued as a puppy; he'd found her wandering around a parking lot late at night.

Those dogs live with us now. They sleep beside my two youngest kids at night. Nya snores underneath my chair as I conduct podcast interviews and write.

This virus is far from gone. The vast implications are still unknown and, tragically, many more families will be affected. That's why I'm donating my advance and all proceeds of this book to the Susan Felice Owens Program for COVID-19 Vaccine Research at Mount Sinai Health System. In the meantime, I hope everyone will remember to wear masks, stay six feet apart, and follow the ever-changing health recommendations.

I hope the following essays by truly sensational, insightful, and talented writers, all of whom have been guests on my podcast, serve as an antidote to the uncertainty and chaos that terrorize our world. That is, if you find time to read them. I hope you will.

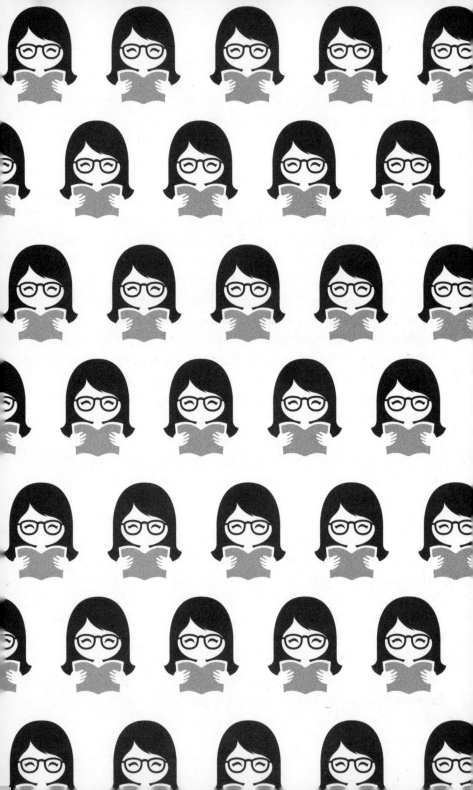

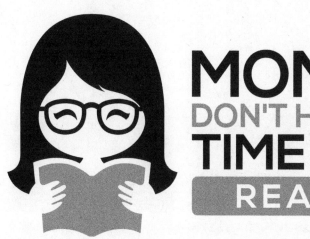

MOMS
DON'T HAVE
TIME TO
READ

Sheltering with Ghosts

ESTHER AMINI

***What would my parents have made of our
locked-down world?***

I'm quarantined with cans of lentil soup, rolls of Bounty, and an assortment of disinfectants just as my memoir *Concealed* is launched into our locked-down world.

As I'm held hostage by the coronavirus, I often think of my Jewish parents who came from the Iranian city of Mashhad and grew up hiding, both physically and emotionally. They concealed their true identity and led duplicitous lives. As underground crypto-Jews, they pretended to be other than who they were in order to survive in a community intolerant of those who were different. Mom stepped out into open-air markets, masked, veiled from head to toe behind a black *chador* as my father prayed from the Koran in public squares, each posing as Muslim. Within the secrecy of their home they were devout Jews. The outside world felt lethal, not because of a widespread virus but due to life-threatening anti-Semitism, a deadly pandemic of its own. After World War II, my parents immigrated to the United States, where I was born, but also hauled with them medieval Mashhad into our New York City home.

Since Iran's societal values were diametrically opposite to America's, so much was misunderstood, and often lost in translation. When my Persian mother spotted bare-armed teens flaunting tattooed biceps she'd belt out "Jinko-lo-vinski,"—her best attempt at "Juvenile Delinquents!" Mom was convinced public reproach would bring about social reform. Thanks to her indecipherable English, our lives were spared. She didn't understand them, nor they her.

But I, too, didn't feel understood. Growing up, I found myself caught between two worlds, the Iranian *chador* and freewheeling America. I was trapped amid the Persian expectation that I be submissive and married by age sixteen, and my wish to break out into the world, unrestricted, and speak.

Growing up, I found myself caught between two worlds, the Iranian *chador* and freewheeling America.

Today, in the midst of a twenty-first-century plague, we're each cooped up, burrowed in our homes, afraid of proximity: especially the breath, sweat, and touch of strangers. And whenever we dare step out, our faces are fully masked. What would Mom say if she were here today, weathering our times? Knowing her, she'd probably jut out her chest, grip her wide Persian hips, and in Farsi bellow, "they will definitely discover a coronavirus vaccine. But it's about time they come out with a vaccine that stops the spread of anti-Semitism!"

And what would be Pop's response, given how terrified he was of people, mail, and all that entered his antiseptic, anti-American abode? He had already perfected "sheltering in place" by avoiding crowds, company, and all forms of human contact. Would he now dig deeper into silence and distrust the outside world even more than he already did?

If my parents were alive with me now wearing face masks and practicing social distancing, memories of their sequestered, underground lives in Mashhad would certainly surface. Unlike Pop, who craved silence and solitude—his aphrodisiac—my boisterous and disobedient mother's insatiable hunger for company would send her breaking out onto city streets. Patience was not her strong suit. I can imagine her scrambling down Fifth Avenue in search of people to stop, see, and gab with. Mom's inner rebel always ruled.

I can't say I identify strongly with either one of my parents. Born in the States, I've been shielded from the kind of dehumanizing terror my parents endured. I'm not hermetic like my father, nor outrageously titanic like my mother. In addition, since I was raised in New York City, my associations with hiding behind locked doors to protect myself from this pandemic are also quite different.

For me, isolation is a gift that favors art. For many, it provides the much-needed climate to invent: compose music, write books, paint, sculpt, think. The creative process flourishes under these circumstances. It demands looking inward and detachment from the outside world, entering one's interior life and getting lost there. And eventually, with determination, pulling out what's buried inside.

> If my parents were alive with me now wearing face masks and practicing social distancing, memories of their sequestered, underground lives in Mashhad would certainly surface.

This is prime time to be undistracted by the comings and goings, the clutter of our modern lives. This is time for reflection. Time to think and not to run. Time to consolidate and evaluate.

For me, it's time to write. Whether I have two hours to pen a thought or two minutes, what's most gratifying is reaching into my silent, overlooked side and letting it speak freely in ways it was not encouraged to do growing up.

It's time, too, to think about the past and be grateful that I am only held hostage temporarily, unlike my parents, who were held hostage by the world they left behind their entire lives.

🕐

Esther Amini is an artist, psychotherapist, and author of the debut memoir Concealed.

The Short Stories I Found in the Sweater Box

CHRIS BOHJALIAN

When I was cleaning out my father's home after he died, I came across a sweater box under his bed. In it were some of the short stories I had written in the third and fourth grade. For a few minutes I sat on the floor and read them, recalling the bedroom in Connecticut in which I had penned them decades earlier, my teachers, and the inspirations for the tales. A couple of times I had to blink back tears, because here was one more indication of how very much my parents had loved me: My mother had saved these stories for years, and then, after she died in 1995, my father had preserved them.

Now, it's also possible that I was on the verge of crying because the stories were absolute train wrecks. Nowhere in them could I find what a creative writing professor might generously have called *promise*. (I must admit, I did take a little pride in my penmanship. My lettering would have made a medieval monk proud.)

But I was struck by how I could see, even in that "apprentice work," two themes that would resonate in my novels as an adult: heartbreak and dread. When my books work—and heaven knows they do not *always* work—those are the points on the narrative compass that matter most. The stories ranged from a tale of a disembodied hand emerging from a wishing well to one about sibling rivalry on the school bus safety patrol. Another ended with this sentence: "The dripping stopped and the vultures had their meal."

There's often a deep connection for writers between what we read for pleasure and what we write. It's not always direct: it's not as if novelists known for writing horror only read horror. (On the other hand, one piece of advice I often give fledging writers is this: write the sort of thing you love to read most. If you love science fiction, write that. If you savor what we call literary fiction, let those books be your inspiration.)

But I know that Esther Forbes's Revolutionary War saga, *Johnny Tremain*, a novel about a fourteen-year-old apprentice silversmith with a crippling hand injury, influenced what I was writing in third grade. I still recall the last line with all of its metaphoric gravitas: "A man can stand up."

Likewise, one week in fourth grade when I was home sick from school, I devoured Shirley Jackson's *The Haunting of Hill House*, a ghost story that to this day scares the hell out of me. I'm sure at nine years old I missed Eleanor Vance's emotional instability and the sadness of her adulthood prior to joining the ghost hunters at Hill House, but I have never forgotten the riveting scene when she jumps from her bed in the night and cries out to her roommate, Theodora, "God! God!—Whose hand was I holding?"

Those two books for me were all about my dual lodestars of heartbreak and dread. To this day, that is what I seem to crave in my reading, whether all is right with the world or we are living in one of those moments in history that we will look back on and think to ourselves, "I know exactly where I was when . . ." I recall finishing Howard Frank Mosher's *A Stranger in the Kingdom* on the front steps of my home in Vermont on a carefree Saturday afternoon in June, the sky cloudless and cerulean, savoring the wistfulness that washed over me and made no sense given the kind of day it was. When I read

Harper Lee's *To Kill a Mockingbird* aloud to my daughter when she was in third grade, we were both a little unmoored by the quiver in my voice as I read the last page—and especially when it broke on that last paragraph:

"He turned out the light and went into Jem's room. He would be there all night, and he would be there when Jem waked up in the morning."

We still have a totemic connection to books made of paper. I love audiobooks on my phone and on occasion I have even read novels on a device. But most books I read are hardcovers or paperbacks. My fiction is alphabetized by author, but I actually have a special section in my library for those books that left me feeling a little broken and a little fragile when I turned the last page—because those are my favorites. Those are the ones I have, on occasion, read two and three and even four times.

Sometimes I wonder what my parents thought when they perused those stories their son had written as a boy. Did they worry about the darkness in them? The sadness? I wasn't a melancholic child. I'm not a morose adult. But then I remind myself that my mother was an avid—almost ferocious—reader; I still have her editions of some of her favorite novels. She probably saw in my short stories the books and movies that had triggered them. She very likely understood that, whether it's *Grimm's Fairy Tales* or *Tales from the Crypt*, children are often drawn to fiction that touches the darkest recesses of the soul.

To this day, that is what I seem to crave in my reading, where all is right with the world or we are living in one of those moments in history that we will look back on and think to ourselves, I know exactly where I was when . . .

And so mostly when I look at those handwritten stories, the blue ink on the white lined paper, I recall that among the great gifts my loving parents gave me was a love of reading in the first place.

◷

Chris Bohjalian is the #1 New York Times *bestselling author of* Midwives *and* The Flight Attendant, *among many other books. His most recent bestselling novel,* The Red Lotus, *was published in March 2020.*

How David Sedaris Is Helping Me Get By

ALLI FRANK

Searching for humor in a most sobering time.

'm currently serving as our house's coronavirus distance learning warden, and my sixth grader and third grader have been asking me for math help in surround sound. With each ticking week, their suspicions that I am in fact clueless, as well as embarrassing, are confirmed. The three of us sit within yelling distance of one another so I'm at the ready for support, but typically my mind is elsewhere.

Back when we thought this whole homeschooling thing would last two weeks max, I ordered pens and pencils in bulk. Some were for now, but most were to be saved for the next school year (I'm a planner). Where the hell have they all gone? Somehow we start every school day with the same declaration: "I need a pen." And my oldest daughter wants intricately braided hairstyles every day for her Google Meet classes, but I cannot, for the life of me, create a straight part. The back of her head looks like tire tracks fishtailing on a road of fresh snow.

Since I was failing my girls as a hairstylist, algebra teacher, and school supplies commissary, and my creative ability to work on my next novel has been zilch, I signed up for David Sedaris's MasterClass. Now, when my daughters ask me for help on any subject, I can point to my screen, then my earbuds, and yell slowly, "I'm in class, too!" For a couple of kids, a middle-aged man sitting in a tweed uphol- stered chair fidgeting with his blazer lapels looks supremely boring, so they truly believe I, too, am on learning lockdown.

And actually, I am. In the first five minutes of my storytelling class, David Sedaris promises all things are funny, eventually. I want to believe him, but I can't help wondering if a pandemic is a statistical outlier. A rogue data point. Will there ever be a time when the story of how coronavirus killed over 100,000 Americans[1] and ushered in uncertainty, fear, and anxiety into every home around the globe becomes funny? And I mean "funny ha-ha," not "funny now pass me another sleeve of shortbread Girl Scout cook- ies." At the moment, it feels unfathomable.

> David Sedaris promises all things are funny, eventually. I want to believe him, but I can't help wondering if a pandemic is a statistical outlier.

I grieve for my life three months ago, loved ones I can't see right now, a stable economy not a fragile one, and hopeful dreams not dashed ones. My focus ebbs and wanes; right now I can barely binge- watch anymore: I was fifteen minutes into a hydrating mask and *Little Fires Everywhere* and I somehow just lost my shit. It's no small task to angry cry when your face is caked in dried mud.

But David (Mr. Sedaris feels too formal after staring at his mug for hours on end) provides some clear and actionable guidance. He offers an obvious tip for storytellers that's often overlooked when the world is operating at full speed and the to-do list is long: be a great observer. When you purposefully observe life, compelling stories and acute details crawl up and settle into your lap. And then you are moved to write. And right now, after two months of creative paral- ysis, I need to get my ass in gear and get a sentence, any sentence,

---

1   Number at time of original publication.

down. So, taking a page from my kids' distance learning lessons and David's instruction, I decide to give myself over to the purposefully observant way of life. As a thought experiment, I imagine I'm in a spring of witnessing and feeling, and I really start to pay attention to detail in this radically bizarre time.

I notice I have four open jars of cinnamon in the cabinet. I find a stash of Halloween candy far back in the closet of my husband's office when I claimed to be "deep cleaning." (All the Twix are now in my sock drawer.) I'm more aware than ever of my inherited runny nose that kicks in if I walk at a crisp clip from the parking lot to the produce aisle at the super-market. (I'm the new Safeway social pariah.) Rolling the bottom of my feet over my kid's lacrosse ball is kind of like a pedicure minus the paint job. Wearing Lycra in a pandemic for a month straight did me no favors when I finally put on jeans. Even with the time to weed, the desire still lags. And somehow every day feels like Sabbath, so I've ended up baking a lot of challah loaves.

When you purposefully observe life, compelling stories and acute details crawl up and settle into your lap.

Oddly, I've never loved my kids and my husband more—it's won-derful. But I'm eager for the day they irritate me again like a low-grade eczema rash. Maybe, just maybe, it's not too soon to laugh?

🕒

Alli Frank, with her coauthor Asha Youmans, is the author of the debut novel Tiny Imperfections.

Wait, Did I Kill My Book Club?
RACHEL LEVY LESSER

After I left, everything just fell apart.

'm not sure how I got in. My friend started her book club almost a decade ago and hand-picked each member. She said she wanted to put together a group of interesting women who would actually read the books and come to meetings ready to discuss them and not just drink wine and talk about our kids and gossip. It was an honor to be nominated!

Being in a book club seemed very on brand for me. I've always loved to read going as far back as my childhood obsession with Ramona Quimby. I devoured most of the books I was assigned in high school and college literary classes, making notes in the margins with pencil to make it seem like I had some kind of insight if the teacher called on me.

At its height, our book club had ten members in total. Everyone who showed up to the meetings had in fact read the book and came prepared with thoughtful questions, unique opinions, and valid points that I hadn't considered on my own. One time, a book club member couldn't make it to the meeting in person so she called in with her notes and we listened to her on speakerphone. We had a few visiting authors come to meetings. We were legit.

Of course we drank wine and talked about our kids and gossiped. It was inevitable, even with the best of intentions. I never minded that part. I knew some of the women in the book club before we became a club and others I met because of it. One member, who I didn't know before, became a close friend.

I discovered new authors and even a new genre (I think!) when we read *The Wilder Life*—about a woman retracing Laura Ingalls Wilder's pioneer journey from the *Little House on the Prairie* days. We tackled a lot of historical fiction spanning most of the nineteenth and a big chunk of the twentieth centuries. We got stuck on World War II for a little longer than I would have liked, but nonetheless, we prevailed. We read memoirs and contemporary fiction, a bit of fantasy, and even some YA. I still think about several of the stories a decade later.

But six years into my book club tenure, I began to lag behind on finishing the books. Reading them started to feel less like something I wanted to do and more like something I had to do—kind of like getting through French in college, *The English Patient* in the movie theater, and geometry in tenth grade. I found myself staying up late to try and finish the books before our next meeting, but I wasn't always successful. I skipped a couple times because I hadn't done the reading.

With my own work deadline looming, my book club reading fell by the wayside. I felt guilty and then stressed out in a weird way which I hadn't felt since being in school. I knew it was time for me to quit, but I really prided myself on not being a quitter.

> Six years into my book club tenure, I began to lag behind on finishing the books. Reading them started to feel less like something I wanted to do and more like something I had to do.

I sent out a very non-me email to the other members quite bluntly saying that I would be leaving the book club. I gave no specific reason why, no excuses, no self-deprecating humor, and not even my usual smiley face emojis or xoxo signature. I heard back from a couple of people asking what was going on. Was I okay? What was the deal?

I gave my fellow book club members a laundry list of everything holding me back, which I fully recognized was annoying because we were all busy. It occurred to me then that reading books that other people assigned to me was not anywhere near the top of my want-to-do list. I wrote that I felt horrible about dropping out, that I knew I was so lame, but that I still wanted to stay in touch about the books they were reading and maybe I could even pop in on a meeting once in a while.

And then, the book club ended.

It never met again. Some said it died. Others said I killed it. It became a running joke among my friends and our spouses. I fully took the blame. Maybe the book club's time had come. Maybe I did everyone a favor. Maybe everyone wanted out for a lot longer than I did. Maybe I was just being honest.

But four years later, I'm still reading. I'm reading what I want to read. These days, that seems to be memoir and contemporary fiction, but that could change. Sometimes I listen to audio books. Sometimes I don't finish the book I started. Sometimes I just listen to an interview with an author on a podcast and call it a day.

It's so incredibly freeing. It actually feels great.

Rachel Levy Lesser is the author of Life's Accessories: A Memoir (and Fashion Guide) *and several other books.*

Ten Unforgettable Mother-Daughter Relationships in Fiction

KELLY McWILLIAMS AND JEWELL PARKER RHODES

(According to two mother-daughter novelists.)

Far too often, mother characters in fiction are absent, dead, or Cinderella-stepmother cruel, because, let's be honest: our culture privileges male wisdom. Patriarchy literally means that valuable goods, including stories and life lessons, mostly pass from father to son.

It's telling that, even now, strong, positive mother-daughter relationships in fiction can be difficult to find. In compiling this list, we were surprised to find ourselves stymied: Didn't Jane Austen write good mothers? Well, Mrs. Dashwood is okay, but Elizabeth Bennet's mom is a ditz! What about *Little Women*? No, Mom, Mrs. March is too perfect to be believable, and everyone knows that one, anyway! Okay, fine. If you're going to have an attitude, I'll take the dogs out instead.

And so on.

(We never said our mother-daughter relationship wasn't fraught!)

But, despite the lack of fictional portrayals, the vast majority of mothers shape their daughters for the better, passing on stories that hold the key to generational mysteries, and sometimes, the strength needed to survive. We've composed this list of books that illustrate mothers that do good—or at least try to—in a believable way. The selections include picture books (as a mother of a three-year-old, sometimes they are the only type of book Kelly has time for), middle-grade novels (gems that stick with you for a lifetime), young adult novels (we love them, enough said!), and a few general fiction selections. We also

Strong, positive mother-daughter relationships in fiction can be a difficult find.

worked hard to find mothers of color in a landscape where the "perfect mother" is often extremely white.

This Mother's Day, we hope you curl up with one of these gorgeous books. And pancakes. Because we wholeheartedly believe each and every mother should receive a healthy stack of homemade pancakes.

1. *Saturday*, Oge Mora

Kelly: I can't remember how this book came into my life, but I'm so glad it did. First of all, the mother portrayed in the stunning mixed-media illustrations isn't white, or thin, or unbelievable in her perfection. She's a regular-sized woman of color trying her best to spend her single day off—Saturday—with her young daughter. As a mother who stays home half-days, it was really interesting to explain to my own daughter that staying home is a privilege, not a right. She's only three, but this is an ongoing conversation we're going to have. Not all mothers get to spend as much time with their daughters as they'd like, and that's something we've got to change. The book is also poignant because, with everything riding on this one day, the mother completely falls apart at the end. Her daughter reminds her: "The day doesn't have to be perfect. We just have to spend it together."

2. *One Crazy Summer*, Rita Williams Garcia

Jewell: *One Crazy Summer* is a terrific book about a less-than-perfect mother-daughter relationship. After being abandoned by her mother, Delphine gains insight into her mother's artistic life and learns that her mother was also abandoned at an early age. It sends the message that it's never too late for mothers and daughters to repair their relationship—which I love.

3. *Beloved*, Toni Morrison

Kelly: Read this book before you're a mom, then read it again after and, lo and behold, it is not the same book! *Beloved* devastated me (think: flattened by a semitruck) when I finally reread it this year, as a mother. Because the hard truth is motherhood depends to a ferocious extent on social context. It is crucial that we remember the sacrifices that mothers were forced to make during times of slavery and Reconstruction, and it is also crucial to compare and make connections to all sorts of hardships that we still face in present day. Moms will feel *Beloved* in their core.

4. *A Big Mooncake for Little Star*, Grace Lin

Jewell: I received an early galley of this sweet, beautiful picture book, and I immediately sent it to my daughter and granddaughter! In the story, Little Star and her mother bake a mooncake and set it "in the sky to cool." Sweet Little Star can't help but sneak out of bed to take a nibble—night after night. Soon enough, and like the moon itself, the mooncake is gone. I love that Lin's story paints the mother-daughter relationship, so often minimized and maligned, on a cosmic scale.

We worked hard to find mothers of color in a landscape where the "perfect mother" is often extremely white.

5. *Our Bodies, Ourselves*, Judy Norsigan

Jewell: Curveball! This book isn't fiction, but it contains the stories of so many women, told in their own voices, that it almost reads like it at times. *Our Bodies, Ourselves* was a revolutionary book when I was a teenager because it dared to address sexuality and coming-of-age from a woman's perspective. I felt honored to be able to share it with my daughter.

6. *When You Know What I Know*, Sonja Solter

Kelly: This middle grade novel-in-verse tells a devastating but important story about child sexual abuse. After the protagonist, Tori, is abused, she tells her mom what has happened, and her mother doesn't believe her, at least not at first. After her mother makes peace with the unimaginable, she becomes a powerful advocate for her daughter, and the two repair their relationship in one of the most moving scenes I've ever read in a fiction piece. As a mother myself, I recognized the mother's mistakes and found them tragically relatable. It's a true work of art, and, despite the heavy topic, a joy to read.

7. *Crazy Rich Asians*, Kevin Kwan

Jewell: *Pride and Prejudice* set in Singapore? Yes, please!

Kelly: Right? My favorite thing about this book (and now also a movie) is that it pays such close attention to the relationship between Rachel and the mother figures in her life: her sharp-tongued mother-in-law, whom she can't possibly impress, and her own mother, who comes to the rescue when all is lost. By the way, Jewell, I think you came to my rescue after a breakup once or twice.

Jewell: I don't remember that.

Kelly: You did!

Jewell: If you say so . . .

Kelly: Unbelievable.

8. *Ella Enchanted*, Gail Carson Levine

Kelly: Speaking of retellings, *Ella Enchanted* tackles Cinderella in a way that really stuck with me. In the opening of this book, Ella is cursed by a silly fairy (who thinks she's blessing her) to always be obedient. But of course, obedience taken too literally can be a horror.

Jewell: I always tried to teach you to think for yourself.

Kelly: In Levine's book, Ella's mother, though she doesn't live long, finds clever ways to teach Ella how to disobey. It's powerful, because in our society female obedience is so highly prized. And yet, our mothers have the power to tell us not to give an eff—

Jewell: They won't print this if you curse.

Kelly: —about the rules. The way I see it, our job as mothers of daughters is to help them to be as disobedient as possible, while still staying safe.

Jewell: It's like the cultural obsession over thinness. I think it was Naomi Wolf who pointed out that it's about obedience more than it is about appearance.

9. *In Search of Our Mother's Gardens: Womanist Prose*, Alice Walker

Jewell: I didn't know black women wrote books until I was in junior college. As I was struggling to find my voice as a writer of color, this essay collection became a healing balm. The marvelous Alice Walker went in search of other black women writers (unfairly obscured by history) and rediscovered Zora Neale Hurston. It demonstrates that our "mothers" on this earth aren't just biological. Our cultural forbearers matter just as much. Where would we be without Zora? Or Alice, for that matter?

10. *Parable of the Talents*, Octavia Butler

Kelly: Growing up, I was a nerd.

Jewell: Yep.

Kelly: I loved science fiction. And I remember asking you, do black people even write science fiction? Because, if so, where the heck is it?

Jewell: In response to that nonsense, I said two words: Octavia. Butler. (Also, shortly after, many other words, because lots of black folks have been writing science fiction for a very long time. It's just not as famous as it ought to be!)

Kelly: Amen. Octavia Butler's *The Parable of the Sower* changed my life. I consider it directly responsible for my novel coming out this summer. *Parable of the Talents*, the sequel to *Parable of the Sower*, is narrated by a daughter who feels neglected by and in awe of her professor/author mother. And I have to say, it really spoke to me!

Jewell: Though I am a professor, I never neglected you, obviously.

Kelly: Of course not. But I always knew you always had other things going on in your life. And as a mom, so do I! It can be tricky to navigate multiple creations. As a portrait of working motherhood, of artistic motherhood, I can't recommend this book highly enough.

Jewell: Happy Mother's Day, everyone!

Kelly: Happy Mother's Day!

🕐

Jewell Parker Rhodes is the New York Times *bestselling author of, most recently,* Black Brother, Black Brother.

Kelly McWilliams is Jewell's daughter, the mother of a toddler, and the author of Agnes at the End of the World.

Why Moms Really Join Book Clubs

ASHLEY PRENTICE NORTON

I t's common knowledge among women that a book club only comes into its own after everyone stops reading the book. When this happens, there will still be the ritual of picking a selection for the next month. Going to the corner bookstore to buy it, putting it on the top of the stack of books that anchor a bedside table. There will still be the rotation of apartments or houses, the salted or savory offerings depending on who's hosting, and the pairs of shoes abandoned in the entryway.

But despite retaining all of the standard book club guidelines, when women emancipate themselves from actually reading the book, it's a brave new world. Now the discussion can wander, and it does. Not scattered and jittery like YouTube, but a steady looking for realness, depth: like water flowing into the cracks between rocks. Once the purses are settled in the hallway, tucked into chairs and sofas, the talking starts. The group is now deeply connected, a sharing of truths, which might only otherwise occur in the context of family, or a therapist's office. Even though they all still love books, adore reading, this gathering now provides a vitality most didn't even know was missing from their lives. They no longer want a Girls Night Out with matchstick umbrellas poking into blended drinks, shots with tacky names, packs of boys who all want the girl with the best body. They want a Girls Night In.

My book club, which lasted eight years, was comprised of seven women: all mothers of children who attended a tiny preschool in the basement of a church on the Upper East Side of Manhattan. All of us, save one, lived within walking distance of the school. All, save two, went to Ivy League schools. Some of us were already friends when the club started; some of us only knew each other in passing, our children in different sections of the preschool.

And then, after meeting for about five months, everything changed. A woman I had previously found abrasive and smug cracked open *Middlemarch* and attempted to read a passage. I will never forget how badly her hands shook when she held the book. Then she started to cry. My hands flew up and gripped both sides of my neck, a tell that something has resonated with me on the deepest level. I reached over and took the book from her, wanting to be reassuring, but at the same time, not wanting to do a full-on rescue, since we weren't the best of friends. I knew by the empathetic looks on all the faces around me that someone else would quickly jump in.

> As they say, some books change your life. For me, it's the ones I didn't read that made all the difference.

She pulled her knees up to her chest on the deep sofa and admitted with more than a touch of shame that she had been laid off from her job. She had been proud of working for this company. She considered it almost as prestigious as her having gone to Harvard. And we all knew the money she earned there mattered, a lot. Everyone had a suggestion as to what might make her feel better. The advice helped, and it did not. She nodded at each reassurance, cried, nodded at the next one, cried. Nod, cry. Nod, cry. I think all of us were hoping for a more profound healing, a catharsis, but all of our efforts seemed to just acknowledge her sadness, not reduce or soften it. She did seem a bit steadier when she stood up from the couch, picked up her *Middlemarch*, and went to leave. It was earlier than when our book club usually broke, but we knew it would be wrong to stay after she left. She would think we were talking about her, and, of course, we would be.

A month later, at our next meeting, we expected her (if she came at all) to be awkward and shy. It wasn't at all like that. She arrived with the first of us, when she had usually been one of the last. She brought brownies. A first. No one ever showed up with food. The brownies were slightly burnt and impossible to get out of the glass dish, but she didn't seem the least bit embarrassed. Someone brought a small dream catcher for her. This was also a first. No one had ever brought a gift before. I wasn't sure how it would go over. She was not, as far as I knew, at all sentimental or craftsy. But her eyes flickered when she saw it, as if she were checking to make sure it wasn't for someone else. When she was sure it was not, she took it with a sincere "thank you," and tucked it in the bag she had used to bring the brownies. We were supposed to be discussing *Never Let Me Go* that night, but we never got around to it. We sat in the living room and ate charred brownie crumbs, sucking our fingers clean instead of washing them because we didn't want to miss anything.

> We weren't a group of women who became friends, so much as we were a tribe.

Over the eight years of our book club, some highlights of what we went through together: Fathers who passed away (cancer, heart attack). Infidelity (some divorced, some tried again). Shock treatment (one had depression that wouldn't go away). And then, one of us died (forty-six, breast cancer). There were also a lot of great stories, laughter, celebrations, that are always harder to remember.

Then, it ended. Eventually, we all had good reasons to stop coming every month. I run into some of the women, but we rarely make plans. We weren't a group of women who became friends, so much as we were a tribe. I'm still a compulsive reader, but it's now a solitary pursuit, and I like it that way. As they say, some books change your life. For me, it's the ones I didn't read that made all the difference.

⊕

Ashley Prentice Norton is the author of novels The Chocolate Money *and* If You Left.

Read More Books

GRETCHEN RUBIN

We're in the midst of an unprecedented world crisis. For many of us, the most immediate consequence is that we're at home with our families, and we have a lot of time on our hands, and we're worried.

What to do? Read, of course! A book can be a wonderful respite from the anxieties of today.

Of my hundreds of happiness-project resolutions, and of the dozens of habits I've tried to form, one of my very favorites is to read more.

Reading is an essential part of my work, and it forms an important part of my social life—I'm in three (yes, three) book groups. Far more important, reading is my favorite thing to do, by a long shot. I'm not a well-rounded person.

Here are some habits that I've adopted over the years to help me get more good reading done.

1. Quit reading.

I used to pride myself on finishing every book I started. I thought that's what a "real reader" did. No more. Life is short. There are too many wonderful books to read. When I stop reading a book I'm not enjoying, I have more time to read the books I do enjoy. And speaking of that . . .

2. Read books you enjoy.

When I'm reading a book I love—for example, I'm now reading Ruth Franklin's biography *Shirley Jackson: A Rather Haunted Life*—I'm astonished by how much time I find to read. Which is another reason to stop reading a book I don't enjoy. Especially when you're under a lot of stress, you want reading to feel like a pleasure, not a duty. (But see #9.)

3. Watch recorded TV.

It's much more efficient to watch recorded shows, because you skip the commercials and control when you watch. Then you have more time to read. And stop watching TV shows you don't enjoy! (See #1.)

4. Skim.

Especially when reading newspapers and magazines, often I get as much from skimming as I do from a leisurely reading. I have to remind myself to skim, but when I do, I get through material much faster. I also give myself permission to skim any part of a nonfiction book that I don't find interesting.

5. Get calm.

These days, with so much going on, it can be hard to turn our attention away from the news and into the world of a book—but once we do, it's such a respite. I have a sticky note posted in our bedroom that says, "Quiet mind." It's sometimes hard for me to settle down with a book; I keep wanting to jump up and take care of some nagging task or check my news updates. But that's no way to read.

> A book can be a wonderful respite from the anxieties of today.

6. Don't fight my inclinations.

Sometimes I feel like I should be reading one book when I actually feel like reading something entirely different. Now I let myself read what I want, because otherwise I end up reading much less. Lately, I've been wanting to reread, because I find it so comforting to revisit old favorites.

7. Maintain a big stack.

I find that I read much more when I have a pile waiting for me. Right now, I have to admit, my stack is so big that it's a bit alarming, but I'll get it down to a more reasonable size before too long.

8. Choose my own books.

Books make wonderful gifts—both to receive and to give—but I try not to let myself feel pressured to read a book just because someone has given it to me. I always give a gift book a try, but I no longer keep reading if I don't want to.

9. Set aside time to read taxing books.

For *Better than Before*, my book about habit-formation, I tried a new reading habit: "Study." Every weekend, I spend time in "study" reading, which covers books that I find fascinating, but that are demanding, and that I might put down and neglect to pick up again. The kind of book that I really do want to read, but somehow keep putting off for months, even years. Similarly, last year I had the "Summer of Proust" and finally read the novels of *Remembrance of Things Past*. I'd planned to have the "Summer of Virginia Woolf" this year, but given the present situation, I may turn that into the "Spring of Virginia Woolf."

> Maybe you don't love to read, so finding more time to read isn't a challenge . . . the larger point is to make sure you're finding time to do whatever it is that you find fun.

And finally, three more tips from great writers and readers:

10. **Randall Jarrell:** "Read at whim! Read at whim!"

11. **Henry David Thoreau:** "Read the best books first, otherwise you'll find you do not have time."

12. **Samuel Johnson:** "What we read with inclination makes a much stronger impression. If we read without inclination, half the mind is employed in fixing the attention; so there is but one half to be employed on what we read."

Maybe you don't love to read, so finding more time to read isn't a challenge for you. The larger point is to make sure you're finding time to do whatever it is that you find fun. Having fun is important to having a happy life, yet it's all too easy for fun to get pushed aside by other priorities. I have to be careful to make time for reading, or, even though I love to read, I might neglect it.

Also, having fun makes it easy to follow good habits; when we give more to ourselves, we can ask more of ourselves. If reading is a treat for you, it's a good idea to make time for it.

The extraordinary events surrounding COVID-19 have given us an opportunity; it's an opportunity that none of us wants, true, but it's an opportunity nevertheless. By reading, we calm ourselves, expand our minds, keep ourselves engaged and mentally nimble, set a good example for any children who are around—and give ourselves utter pleasure.

⊕

Gretchen Rubin is the five-time New York Times *bestselling author of* The Happiness Project, Happier at Home, The Four Tendencies, Better than Before, *and* Outer Order Inner Calm. *She is the host of award-winning podcast* Happier with Gretchen Rubin.

A Technology Pioneer Shuts Down, Weekly

TIFFANY SHLAIN

O ver a decade ago, I needed a drastic change. Within days of each other, my father died and my daughter was born. These life-altering events made me think about the brevity of our time here, and question how I was spending it. I didn't like where we seemed to be headed, with everyone staring at screens instead of connecting with the people we loved right in front of us.

I needed a revolution to transform the situation, and I found it. For twenty-four hours, my family and I went screen-free. Nearly a decade later, we've done it almost every Saturday since. Establishing a weekly Tech Shabbat is the best decision we've ever made.

Living twenty-four/six feels like magic, and here's why: it seems to defy the laws of physics, as it both slows down time and gives us more of it. I laugh a lot more on that day without screens. I notice everything in greater detail. I sleep better. It strengthens my relationships and makes me feel healthier. It allows me to read, think, be more creative, and reflect in a deeper way. Each week I get a full reset. Afterward, I'm much more productive and efficient, with positive effects that radiate out to the other six days. It even helps renew my appreciation for all that I have access to online, giving me that *Wow, the Internet* realization fresh each week. Who would have thought technology could be more potent in its absence?

> I needed a revolution to transform the situation, and I found it.

28

One day a week without screens improves our children's lives, too. Our daughters, Odessa (sixteen) and Blooma (ten), have done this practice most of their lives, and it has shaped how they interact with technology in extremely beneficial ways. They enjoy their time off screens and look forward to it. It feels like a vacation every week. We all look forward to it with the same anticipation, and it provides that same feeling of deep relaxation we get when we go away.

Because it expands your sense of time, it makes your day off feel like two days in one. Going screen-free once a week is like having a metaphysical remote control, with a pause button for the twenty-four/seven world, that turns your life back on.

The fact that my family has practiced Tech Shabbat for so long surprises people. Ken is a UC Berkeley professor of robotics. I've also spent my career exploring the online world, first by establishing the Webby Awards, then as a filmmaker examining how all this connectedness is changing our lives today and will continue to do so in the future. We're both deeply involved with technology and constantly pushing on its edge. Yet I found great meaning and power in a technology invented several millennia in the past. More than three thousand years ago, the concept of Shabbat (also known as the Sabbath) transformed the world. Before then, time had no pauses: it was day after day after day. Shabbat made it so each week ended with a day off, for everyone, of every social class. The run-on sentence of time got a period, and humankind got a chance to catch its breath and focus.

> I laugh a lot more on that day without screens. I notice everything in greater detail. I sleep better.

All these years later, practicing our version of Shabbat helps my family be present with one another, appreciate the small things, daydream, and get a different viewpoint on living. It encourages resourcefulness and recalls a simpler time. Doing something the same day as others all over the world are doing it also reminds us that we are connected to something larger than ourselves and offers a way to live a more meaningful life. Turning off screens and disconnecting from the online network helps us use tech in a way that prevents tech from using us.

⊕

Tiffany Shlain is the author of 24/6: Giving Up Screens One Day a Week to Get More Time, Creativity and Connection. *An Internet pioneer and Emmy-nominated filmmaker, Tiffany has been honored by* Newsweek *as one of the "Women Shaping the 21st Century."*

Dystopian Fiction Is Made for This Moment

REEMA ZAMAN

**Turning to the frightening genre for
wisdom amid the madness.**

I live alone in an apartment holding only what I need: sunlight, bed, desk, chair, three bookcases, two closets, a refrigerator of food. Every detail tailored to me, purposeful, beautiful, nothing superfluous. I'm told often my space is minimalist, or that I need more furniture, maybe a plant, or a pet.

One bookcase is dedicated to memoir. The second, dystopian literature. The third combines the first two, books like Jonathan Karl's *Front Row at the Trump Show*.

As a young girl in Bangladesh and Thailand, I turned to dystopian fiction for the comforting intimacy of feeling seen and understood, and the *Sweet Valley Twins* and *Baby-Sitters Club* series for escapism. I loved the Twins and Babysitters for their endearing innocence courtesy of American privilege. The key was understanding that their personalities were shaped by their experiences, not mine. This served me well when I immigrated to the United States for college.

I'm now an American citizen, relying again on dystopian favorites. Some books are new, others, revisited through heightened stakes. I'm currently writing a dystopian novel myself, called *Paramita*, which means perfection in Sanskrit. I began writing it in April after learning that a series of lucrative speaking events had been canceled due to the coronavirus; 70 percent of my projected annual income vanished nearly overnight. Fueled by urgency, I turn to my work-in-progress every day to converse with an ensemble of characters that gives me a semblance of human connection. Since I'm quarantined alone, they fortify me. The lens of storytelling is like sunglasses. Without story, my eyes burn from the glare of the world.

> The lens of storytelling is like sunglasses. Without story, my eyes burn from the glare of the world.

A few friends, concerned by my full-body immersion into dystopia, have encouraged lighter fare for comfort or escapism, reasoning that outside my apartment teems a world caught in the maw of the coronavirus pandemic, a racial reckoning, and the Trump administration.

Yet the outside world is precisely why I've turned now to dystopian literature. Anytime I've tried reading a book for escape from our present reality, I get a few lines in, and I feel the way I do when having brunch with people with far more privilege than me: I can don the costume, play the part, mimic the twinkling laughter and airy language, but it's not my natural habitat. The entire time, I long to return home to the voices of my mother tongue.

Those voices are Margaret Atwood, Ursula Le Guin, and Suzanne Collins, who examine humankind's scathing truths with an unflinching gaze: the searing opposite of escapism. I first read Collins's *The Hunger Games* as an ARC in 2007, although back then, I didn't know what an "advanced reader's copy" was. I was twenty-four, a struggling actress in New York, living with eleven flatmates in a converted factory in Chinatown. One flatmate was an assistant publisher at Random House, hence the ARC.

Two pages in, I knew *The Hunger Games* would shake the planet. When the book came out, I bought copies for my family, pleading, "Read this. It's the truth." In 2007 it was dazzling; in 2020, the book lights my brain on fire.

The Hunger Games examines the exploitation of essential workers in the world of Panem through the story of Katniss, a sixteen-year-old girl, a reluctant warrior battling the ruthless President Snow. Katniss comes from the coal-mining District 12, the poorest in the nation. Her weaponry is her bow and arrows, courage and intelligence. The weaponry President Snow wields is his expert use of reality television and militarized government to spread fear, gain power, exert cruelty. Sound familiar?

While the people of Panem actively fight their class divide and oppression, it has taken a combination of a global pandemic, a racial reckoning, and the Trump Administration for many in America to finally acknowledge the systemic injustices that exist in our world.

We live with an infrastructure that rewards people for being white, murders people for being black, and depends upon and exploits essential workers. Dystopian literature like *The Hunger Games* reflects our current realities because our reality is dystopian. It always has been. What is new is our enforced physical and spiritual quarantine; with nowhere else to go or look, life-and-death stakes have forced us to see what we are so we may evolve.

With dystopian literature, the reader looks within and around with boldness and curiosity. We enter a pact with the author that says, "I'm not hiding anything. This is what we may become should we continue in our current manner." It's why memoir and dystopian literature are a perfectly compatible couple residing in my home.

When Atwood describes June's entrapment in *The Handmaid's Tale*, or Collins voices Katniss's rage over a corrupt government, they channel thoughts I've had, sentences I've spoken.

I turn to them now for wisdom amid the madness. Through quarantine, Atwood reminds me that even in the barest of rooms and direst of circumstances, a woman has her resilience. In fact, Katniss adds, it is the bareness of the room, the direness of the earth, that stokes the fire within.

🕐

Reema Zaman is an award-winning speaker, actress, and the author of the debut memoir I Am Yours.

The Books Getting Me through Quarantine

EILENE ZIMMERMAN

The titles I turn to when things fall apart.

I live in New York City's West Harlem neighborhood, and I'm likely going to be here for the duration of this pandemic. My kids are three thousand miles away on the West Coast, and even if—in my panic and fear and motherly anxiety—I wanted to rush to them, I really can't. There are few flights now, for one thing. Driving my ten-year-old Ford Fiesta across the country is not a realistic option, and my kids have small apartments and roommates. And anyway, it would be irresponsible to bring whatever I have or have not been exposed to in New York City out of state during a public health crisis.

Instead, I'm holed up in my apartment, trying to promote my book *Smacked* as best as I can, finishing graduate school, and spending too much time on Twitter. I am trying to meditate each day, in order to get my mind to stop spinning out scenario after scenario (none of them good), to refocus on the fact that I'm here and healthy and loved—and that's something. Really, that's everything.

I'm also constantly reminding myself that control is an illusion. Sure, we can control how we react to things. We can don masks and gloves and plan out a trip to the pharmacy or supermarket; we can put in new rules for kids at home trying to do schoolwork remotely.

We can cram a table into a corner and call it a home office, for now. These are things we do to put some order and structure into our lives, but that's not the same as control. And that lack of control, the not knowing, is what is creating anxiety and despair for so many of us—I should know.

. . . you can plan and plan and plan and then life happens the way it happens . . .

My memoir is about many things, and one of them is that although we think we have a pretty good idea of how things will unfold in our lives, we're usually wrong. My ex-husband and the father of my children died in a way I never anticipated, never in a million years. He was only fifty-one years old, incredibly smart and successful, financially well-off, a partner in a sexy, Silicon Valley law firm, supremely capable. And yet . . . he died on his bathroom floor, an intravenous drug addict.

I was on the phone with my son the other day, a newly minted college graduate now facing a collapsing job market, trying to adjust his expectations of both the near future and the world in general. We were talking about how nothing is turning out the way we thought it would. And I said, "We should know this, we should know this because of what happened to Dad." We reminded each other that yes, you can plan and plan and plan and then life happens the way it happens and the only control we have is in our reaction.

My reaction to the current crisis, as a writer and reader, is a turn toward books—reading and listening to them. I'm reading in two ways. One that lets me escape—books about invented worlds of Greek gods and mythical wars, like *Circe* by Madeline Miller and *The Silence of the Girls* by Pat Barker. I read *The Dirty Life: A Memoir of Farming, Food, and Love* by Kristin Kimball, so I could immerse myself in Kimball's experience of moving from New York City to start a farm on five hundred acres near Lake Champlain. I read—again— my friend Adrienne Brodeur's luscious memoir *Wild Game*, with its mouth-watering descriptions of food and Cape Cod, and I even downloaded the audio book of Tolstoy's *War and Peace*. I mean, why not?

I'm also finishing up a graduate degree in social work and perhaps because of that, or because I was the one to find my ex-husband Peter dead on his bathroom floor, I'm also drawn to books about fear, about death, about grief, and about being present and bearing witness to all of it. I have read and am reading Thich Nhat Hanh's book *Fear: Essential Wisdom for Getting Through The Storm*, Kerry Egan's beautiful book *On Living*, Joan Halifax's *Being with Dying* and *Advice Not Given: A Guide to Getting Over Yourself*, by the Buddhist psychiatrist Mark Epstein.

I'm also listening to podcasts where authors talk about books and tell stories. Yesterday I was listening to the podcast *Everything Happens* hosted by Kate Bowler, author of *Everything Happens for a Reason: And Other Lies I've Loved* (which I just ordered from the adorable shop Skylark Books in Columbia, MO). Bowler was speaking with Sister Helen Prejean, a nun who works with inmates on death row in Louisiana's Angola State Prison. Prejean's well-known book-turned-movie, *Dead Man Walking*, is the story of Patrick Sonnier, an inmate who Prejaen befriended and accompanied on his journey to the electric chair, both physically and spiritually. She recalled for Bowler being the only person permitted to be with Sonnier when he was electrocuted. Sonnier wanted her to leave, didn't want to subject the nun to something so traumatic. But Prejean told Bowler, "All I knew was there's no way this man is going to be electrocuted to death by the state . . . every face looking at him wants to see him die. And I said, 'Pat, I don't know what it's going to do to me, but you look at my face when they do this, and I'll be the face of love for you.'"

> We can use books to help us make sense of things as they are today, and also to help us imagine a brighter future.

In all that beauty I felt such sadness. For the world right now, for the world my kids are inheriting, for my city, and, on a very personal level, for Peter, my ex-husband and friend. He died alone, and I truly believe he so needed that face of love at the end.

Like all good stories, Prejean's is inspirational as well as aspirational. We can use books and stories to help us make sense of things as they are today, and also to help us connect with our higher selves and imagine a brighter future. My reading is helping me understand, every day, the importance of calling friends, seeing them virtually, taking food to my elderly mother and reading to her, making sure everyone in my life knows they are loved. And in turn, knowing I am loved. Because, really, what else is there?

🕐

Eilene Zimmerman is the author of Smacked: A Story of White-Collar Ambition, Addiction, and Tragedy. *She has been a journalist for three decades, covering business, technology, and social issues for national magazines and newspapers, including the* New York Times, *where she was a columnist for many years.*

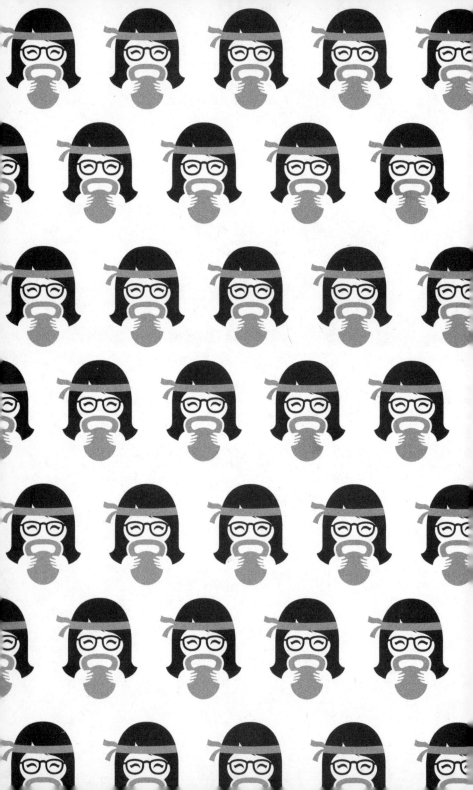

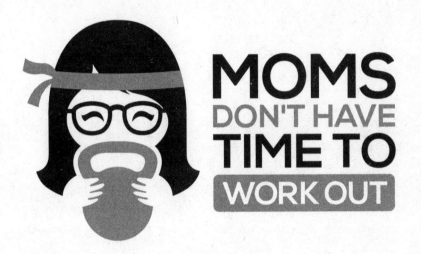

What My Father Taught Me
ELLIOT ACKERMAN

He never held my baggy pants and bad attitude against me.

Everybody knew the color of my boxer shorts, much to my father's chagrin. As a teenager, skateboarding was my passion and sagging pants was the style. Every morning I'd shuffle down to breakfast before school, my belt cinched at an impossible angle around my hips, the backs of my jeans frayed like some tattered battle flag. Taking my seat at the table, I'd wordlessly spoon up my cereal and slurp the sugary milk from the bowl. My parents' redline for academics was no Cs on your report card. I brought home mostly B-minuses. An exception was a D in PE. The teacher noted that I fell asleep in meditation exercises and refused to pull up my gym shorts.

I wasn't a bad teen. I just didn't care. Most of my friends in high school were a year or two older. They dabbled in drugs. They had parties. At the time it felt edgy; in retrospect it was typical kid stuff.

My brother was quite different. He was two years older, but three years ahead of me in school. A mathematical prodigy, he'd skipped a grade and had gone on to study at Harvard where he also wrestled. To my parents' credit, never once did it occur to me that they might be prouder of their Harvard-enrolled collegiate wrestling son than their B-minus-delivering skateboarding son. Toward the end of my junior year, my mother was sorting mail at the kitchen table. Each night

I usually received one or two promotional materials from colleges. One had arrived from the US Air Force Academy. She showed it to me and threw it in a pile to be trashed with the others. "Wait," I said. "Let's keep that one." She set it off to the side, but not before offering a concerned look.

My father could have easily pointed out that I was hardly a prime candidate for one of the highly competitive service academies. Instead, he simply listened.

When my father asked me about it in my room a couple of days later, I told him I was interested in the military, though admittedly I didn't really know what that meant. He could have easily pointed out that my grades weren't great and that I'd never played a single sport. I was hardly a prime candidate for one of the highly competitive service academies. Instead, he didn't hold my saggy pants against me, or my hair, or anything I'd done up until this moment. He simply listened and said, "We should probably get started."

Each of the service academies had a physical fitness test for applicants. I printed it out. I put on my gym shorts (pulling them up to the appropriate place, this time) and went to the local park with my father to see how I scored. Push-ups, sit-ups, and pull-ups were part of the test. I had two minutes to do as many of each as I could. My father had brought a stopwatch, but he wouldn't need it. I couldn't last two minutes at anything. That day in the park, I did eight push-ups, about twenty sit-ups, and couldn't manage a single pull-up.

I brooded over my dinner that night and didn't say much. The following morning, my father had drawn up an exercise routine on a yellow legal pad. He left it by my door.

That summer between my junior and senior year, I followed the instructions on that legal pad religiously. Each day, my father would ask me: "Did you get your workout in?" He wasn't being pushy; he was simply letting me know he cared. Some days we took jogs together, on others he drove me to the gym, but mostly he gave me my space. By the fall, my older group of friends was off at college, and I was singularly focused on heading into the military. By Thanksgiving, when those same friends returned home for the holiday, I was unrecognizable.

That year I lettered in two varsity sports and wound up acing the physical fitness test for the service academies. My transformation was dramatic and complete by the spring, when I was on my way into an officer-commissioning program for the Marines.

I went on to serve eight years in the military in two wars. Today, I'm a father of young children, and when people meet me, I imagine my identity as a veteran is probably what they see first. But it wasn't always there; in fact, my journey was

> Each day, my father would ask me: "Did you get your workout in?" He wasn't being pushy; he was simply letting me know he cared.

an improbable one. Had my father not seen what so few could, it's a journey I likely wouldn't have made.

On Father's Day, I say a little prayer of thanks to him. And I say a little prayer for myself: Through poor grades, saggy pants, and too long hair, may I always see my kids not only as they are, but as they might be.

⊕

Elliot Ackerman served five tours of duty in Iraq and Afghanistan and is the recipient of the Silver Star, the Bronze Star for Valor, and the Purple Heart. He is the author of five books, including the new novel Red Dress in Black & White.

Rowing into Midlife, One Stroke at a Time

KAREN DUKESS

In a single month, I quit my job, became an empty nester, and joined a community rowing team.

f I told you I'd never been on a team before, I'd be lying. I was on a team. For exactly one day in ninth grade. My mother—the same one who'd lovingly stitched me a needlepoint pillow of a snail saying "Don't rush me"—convinced me to get moving and try out for the field hockey team. I was five-foot-two, more spherical than strapping, and during that one afternoon learned that thwacking a ball when running with a hockey stick is surprisingly difficult. Ever since, I've kept a respectable distance from group sports, sticking to my principle that there's no me in team.

Until a year and a half ago. It wasn't a midlife crisis, more a confluence of events in the river of life. In a single month, I'd sold my debut novel, quit my speechwriting job at the United Nations, become an empty nester, and read *The Boys in the Boat.* I suddenly had time—way too much time—in a quiet home office in a quieter suburb. In that context, a small ad for the community Learn to Row program, an ad I'd seen countless times over the past decade, called out to me. With my newfound freedom, the early—and I mean early—morning sessions were not out of the question. And with a great deal of willpower, I chose not to be intimidated by the photo of the strong female rowers in skimpy Lycra singlets.

What did it matter if I was the weakest, the heaviest, or the oldest? I enrolled.

Just like that, I became a member of the Pelham Community Rowing Association. Four mornings a week, I'd report to the boathouse while the mist was still rising from the water. Together with three other newbie women, along with a few experienced rowers who were there to help out, we would carry the boats on our shoulders down to the dock. I learned how to get in the boat, which is not as easy as it sounds, and after a few weeks, managed to get out of the boat without rolling my body onto the dock like a sea lion. I learned the three phases of the rowing stroke—

With burning glutes, a pounding heart, and the sweatiest smile, I felt— for the first time in my life—like I was, maybe, sorta, kind of an athlete.

the catch, the drive, and the recovery—and how to avoid "catching a crab," when the blade gets caught awkwardly in the water, sometimes so forcefully that the rower is catapulted from the boat.

With the careful instruction of our preternaturally patient coach, Chris, I learned to propel the boat with my legs and mirror the stroke of the rower in front of me without looking at her oars. Day after day, as Chris instructed us through a bullhorn from his launch boat, we learned to row together. Though we may not have become "a poem of motion, a symphony of swinging blades" like those boys in the boat, we sometimes found a rhythm, at least for a little while, and experienced the boat-bound thrill of slicing the lagoon like a knife.

I was in it for the outdoor season when I signed up. The indoor winter rowing machine workouts struck me as all the misery with none of the misty beauty. But by the time the season was over, I'd grown attached to my boat mates. And I wanted to continue to get stronger and better. I signed on for the winter season, and even started to like rowing on a stationary "erg," probably because I was doing it as part of a team and with a coach.

About six weeks into our erg sessions, Chris started talking about the club's annual indoor regatta, when rowers in various categories compete on ergs in a 2000-meter race, about 1.25 miles. Four of the other women signed up right away. I hesitated. There was an extremely good chance I'd be the slowest in the women-over-fifty category. Who wanted to volunteer to come in last?

I wasn't having a midlife crisis, it was more of a confluence of events in the river of life.

But the more I shared my fears with my teammates, the more I realized that no one cared about how fast I went except for me. It's often said that women feel invisible when they get older, and that can be painful. But on the flip side, getting older can free you from worrying about what other people think. And the truth was, the more I got used to my plan, the more eager I became to see if I could execute it. Two days before the regatta, I signed up.

The morning of, I drove to a school gym in the Bronx, a trip I'd made countless times to watch my sons play basketball. Now, my palms were the sweaty ones. I hopped on an erg beside my rowing pals and together we warmed up and then made that middle-aged-female, last-minute dash to the restroom. When it was time for our bracket, we wished each other luck and went to our assigned ergs.

Two thousand meters is simultaneously an endurance event and a sprint. I never once glanced at the race board to check my standing. I kept my eyes focused on my erg's computer screen, on pace with a 2.22 split, my goal of two minutes and twenty-two seconds per five hundred meters. I made my time, to the tenth of a second.

And I came in last. With burning glutes, a pounding heart, and the sweatiest smile, I felt—for the first time in my life—like I was, maybe, sorta, kind of an athlete.

The endorphins carried me through that week. And the next, when the talk back in the studio was all about the threat of a pandemic. And then, three weeks after the regatta, I finished a workout feeling chilled. The next day, I tested positive for the coronavirus. By the end of the week, our boathouse was off-limits. The park where it's located was turned into a testing site. As I slowly recovered, self-quarantined, rowing wasn't even on my radar.

Now it's spring and perfect rowing weather—sunny, cool, only the tiniest breeze. As I wait to hear when rowing will start again, I can't help but reflect on all the real barriers the pandemic has thrown in our way. What a waste it is to be held back by obstacles of our own making, fears of how silly we'll look or how we'll compare to others. One day life will resume again, and there will be glorious new failures to pursue—if we let ourselves.

Karen Dukess is a former speechwriter and the author of the debut novel The Last Book Party, *now available in paperback.*

Want to Stop Comparing Yourself to Others? Try Tree Pose

JAN ELIASBERG

How yoga finally helped me silence my nagging inner voice.

I've been practicing yoga for twenty-five years. I know this precisely because I took my first class when I was pregnant with my now twenty-four-year-old daughter.

I was not one of those blissed-out pregnant yoga mamas. I was cranky and hyper-focused on all the things my bloated body, my bulging tummy, and my swollen feet wouldn't let me do. I'd been a Type A exerciser, pounding the pavement and sweating like a sinner in church. I liked the challenge of a really tough workout. But loss of cartilage in my knee combined with twenty pounds of pregnancy weight ruled out that kind of exercise. So when my pregnant neighbor asked me to go to a prenatal yoga class with her, I couldn't find a reason to refuse.

As I waddled into that first class I inwardly rolled my eyes at the sylph-like women with luminous skin and not an ounce of body fat, holding their tiny, perfectly rounded bumps like expensive accessories while twisting their limbs into impossible poses. But still I went back the next day, and then the next.

The class would begin with everyone announcing her name and due date. And almost every day there would be an empty space in the circle of yoga mats; one very pregnant woman would be gone, only to reappear a couple of weeks later with a newborn for the class to coo over. Soon, the familiar faces of my due date cohort disappeared. My neighbor's due date arrived and two days later she wasn't in class; her husband called the next day to tell us they'd had a boy.

> As I waddled into that first class I inwardly rolled my eyes at the sylph-like women with luminous skin and not an ounce of body fat . . .

My due date came and went. A week later, the teacher herself could barely conceal her concern. I was already scared about labor, but my classmates' free-floating anxiety made it infinitely worse.

Finally, after a nudge from my ob/gyn and thirty-six hours of labor, Sariel arrived scarlet-faced and screaming into the world. In the aftermath, my body was bruised and I could barely stand up to push the stroller down the street. But remarkably, I missed yoga. As soon as I could walk, I went right back. I almost couldn't help it—I was addicted to the total sense of contentment and ease I felt at the end of class.

Everything that yoga addicts proselytize about is true: Your muscles become longer and leaner; your skin looks better, and day-to-day crankiness becomes the exception rather than the rule.

Here's what they don't tell you:

That chattering, nasty little voice in your head that constantly compares your body with other women's bodies finally shuts the hell up. I no longer hear the distracting static of my brain insisting that I have to lose five pounds before I'll really be okay. All I think about when I'm on my mat is how grateful I am that my body can achieve these remarkable shapes, or some approximation thereof.

You will also have fuller and more complete access to your emotions. The amount of effort and stress it takes to keep feelings under the surface starts to ebb away, leaving nothing but the feeling. Many is the time I've burst into tears in a yoga class; no one gives me dirty looks, they've all been there, too. The teacher might come over and put a gentle hand on my back or might just let me cry until I'm all cried out. It's a glorious feeling of release.

I no longer hear the distracting static of my brain insisting that I have to lose five pounds before I'll really be okay.

In yoga you practice all the skills you start to lose as you age: Tree pose improves your balance; pigeon pose improves your flexibility, and chaturanga dandasana (holding plank or push-up position) is fabulous for bone density. Strength, flexibility, and balance—those aren't just the skills we need for aging gracefully, they're the skills we need for living gracefully.

They are also wonderful skills to practice during the COVID-19 pandemic. Rolling out that yoga mat marks a time and space for a ritual that feels sacred. Whether I'm live-streaming a class, playing a prerecorded class with one of my favorite teachers in a subscription series, or just moving through opening asanas on my own, everything in the outside world always melts away.

Concerns about my daughter living with friends in Brooklyn fade. Panic about book sales dissipates. And loneliness, the most difficult part of this self-quarantine, is redefined as peaceful solitude.

Jan Eliasberg is a director, screenwriter, and author of the debut novel Hannah's War.

After My Daughter Died, My Son Took Up Rock Climbing

SUZANNE FALTER

One slip, one mistake, and my last remaining child would be gone.

Not long ago, my son Luke sent me a video from his first climb in the Sierra Nevada. The video shows him breathless, paused on the side of a mountain wall, eleven thousand feet above the ground. He shouts, "ahoy there!" and points to his climbing partner's sliding-X anchor, noting that it's not redundant. "Luckily, my mom doesn't know what redundancy means," he says with a laugh.

No, but Mom has Google, and Mom found out.

According to *Climbing: From Gym to Rock*, an anchor that is "not redundant" means there is nothing to back it up if it were to fail. One slip, one mistake, and my last remaining child would fall to his death. Luke reminds me that he is a certified professional climbing guide. Still, I worry.

Not long after his sister Teal's sudden death in 2012, Luke decided to become a serious rock climber—the sort who climbs thousands of feet at a time and dreams of working for Yosemite Search and Rescue. He's twenty-four, an adventurer with a wild mountain spirit, a sharp mind, and nerves of steel. And he scares me to death. I once asked Luke if his desire to take up such a dangerous sport had anything to do with Teal's death.

"Yeah, something like that," he said. And I have to admit, that makes sense. After all, there is something strangely freeing about a massive life upheaval. When life shakes you to the core and you're reduced to rubble, the things you value most become abundantly clear. Suddenly, there is no holding back from what you love, just as there is no more wasting time on things that hardly matter. Life gets pulled into a swift, clear order that you can't un-see.

Teal knew this secret long before she died. She was an epileptic born with a deep and passionate love for travel. Armed with her meds, she made her way fearlessly around the world, traveling mostly alone with a backpack. And she did this even though she suffered a grand mal seizure on a beach in Ghana, and another near seizure in a hostel in Marrakech. Whenever she had enough dollars in her pocket from waitressing, she'd suddenly be off again, flying off to Dublin or Bangkok.

> When life shakes you to the core and you're reduced to rubble, the things you value most become abundantly clear.

Though she died at the impossibly young age of twenty-two, Teal managed to wander around most of the continents. It was, quite simply, what she had to do. "Mom, seriously—my epilepsy is no big deal," she'd insist.

This is the same voice Luke uses when he says, "Mom, seriously—climbing is incredibly safe." It's that all-knowing voice of unreason, the one you hear loudly when you're, say, under thirty. Yet, it's also the voice of unbridled desire. And it's the one I have to heed if I'm going to get along in this life.

Still, I worry for Luke, just as I worried every time Teal headed off to farm in Belgium or to backpack through Southeast Asia. How could I not? When my daughter was alive, there was always a phantom rapist in my imagination who would pick her up on some back road in a country where she couldn't speak the language. My imagination would stew for days about a possible terrorist attack on a train, or a collision when she was off riding a bike somewhere. It didn't help that Teal resolutely refused to wear a medical ID bracelet, just as she was reluctant to tell the various roommates she lived with about her epilepsy.

Ultimately, these children of ours have to grow up to do what they're going to do, whether it suits us or not.

Her philosophy was *nunc vitae*. Life is now. In other words, quit worrying and get on with it.

As it turned out, Teal did have a few close calls, including being hit by a car while riding a bicycle in Texas, and talking her way out of a near rape in Thailand. But each time she walked away unscathed. And each time she didn't tell me about it until much later.

You could say that Teal prepared me for Luke's high adventure streak. These days, when he's not climbing, he's skiing trees in the subzero backcountry. At night. With a headlamp. Or he's pursuing his other hobby, working in the back of an ambulance hurtling through Vermont's frozen, snowy roads. Last Christmas, I gave him a cheery tea towel that says, "Every day do something to terrify your family." He liked that gift.

I try to keep in mind something I learned when Teal was in Ghana as a seventeen-year-old. She was there, ostensibly, to teach English, but really she was there to quench her ceaseless thirst for global connection. One night, I called her when it was well past 11:00 p.m., and her hostess answered the phone. Maria was a generous, large-hearted Ghanaian whose business it was to sit all day long in her plastic chair in front of her house, greeting her neighbors and looking after the girls who stayed with her. Though our lives were vastly different, she had some sterling advice for me. When she told me that Teal was out with her friends, I got alarmed.

"But it's well past eleven!" I protested. Maria gave a long, warm laugh.

"Oh, mama," she chuckled. "You worry too much."

There you have it. Ultimately, these children of ours have to grow up to do what they're going to do, whether it suits us or not. They have to make good choices and bad choices and in between choices, and we are left to soothe, when necessary. Mostly, we're just meant to cheer them on.

Should I have been more protective of Teal? Should I have somehow anticipated she might suddenly drop dead, even though I never knew such a thing was even possible? No and no. This is the messy, uncertain, awkward, and difficult flow of life. Sometimes it's just plain heartbreaking.

In the end, Teal's death had nothing to do with her adventure streak. She had a cardiac arrest in a locked bathroom in her San Francisco apartment. The cause will never be known, though it is possible she suffered from a rare condition called Sudden Death in Epilepsy, which randomly strikes one in a thousand epileptics.

So life goes on. Luke runs up mountains until he dry heaves, and I watch from a distance, fiercely loving him. I let go, trusting him and his mad desires, just as I once trusted Teal's. Twenty years ago, I watched him climb everything he could find, including the poles on the IRT while it rattled along at high speed. Just as I let him climb then, I must let him climb now.

Suzanne Falter is an author, speaker, and host of the podcast Self-Care for Extremely Busy Women. *Her many nonfiction books include* The Extremely Busy Woman's Guide to Self-Care *and* The Joy of Letting Go.

I Don't Want to Work Out.
I'm a Lorelai

CHRISTINA GEIST

Here's the truth: I have very little interest in working out, at home or anywhere else, despite the fact that I now have plenty of time.

In my 1980s childhood, my mom drank Tab and Diet Coke but cooked us real, homemade, healthy meals every night. Many parents smoked in my generation, and few walked around in workout clothes all day, but we all turned out just fine. I don't know if moms had time to work out in my youth. Even if they had the time, they just didn't. Judging by the TV moms I loved most, Alice Keaton, Carol Brady, and "Ma" from *Little House on the Prairie*, not a single American mom burned a calorie before Jane Fonda released her first tape.

Fast-forward to 2020. Here I am. A mom in a generation of maxed-out moms. I've been burning the candle at both ends since well before the quarantine. I was raised to have it all, with no glass ceiling. As a result, I have been actually trying to do it all, as in *all* of it, while maintaining a solid marriage, a strong core, a balanced diet, and some kind of mindfulness practice.

Here I am now. A mom in the quarantine era. Figuring out how to manage my newfound anxiety while continuing to run two small businesses, while homeschooling two kids, once we get through these two weeks of "spring break" and it's no longer acceptable for them to spend the day with Bart Simpson.

Here I am now. Worrying about my kids' physical activity levels while suddenly inundated with images of my fellow moms working out more than they did before. There's my friend teaching a yoga class by Zoom. There's my husband clicking into the same Peloton I used to prop up my phone while on Instagram. There are my home weights, sitting on my nice little home yoga mat, gathering dust.

I don't know if moms had time to work out in my youth. Even if they had the time, they just didn't.

Here I am now. Certainly thinking about working out. But, somehow, not doing it. It's not that I don't want to work out. It's not that I don't have the time. I have plenty of time. It's just that I will prioritize almost anything else that can be considered "work" over working out.

My days go something like this:

8:00 a.m.: I wake up. I put on workout clothes.

9:00 a.m.: I go to my desk, and sit down and do work, in my workout clothes.

12:00 p.m.: I take a break from work. But, instead of working out, I find myself toasting two slices of rye bread so the cheese will melt perfectly over my turkey. I add the mayo and a side of barbecue chips, while still in my workout clothes.

3:00 p.m.: I have a break from work. This is a natural time to work out. Yet, I have this uncanny ability to find other "work" to do instead. I proceed with dusting the bookshelves and organizing the books by height and color, showing my daughter how to make a photo album (remember those?), going to put laundry in and then completely reorganizing the entire laundry room and cleaning supply cabinet, realizing then that I could iron that pile of napkins, and then passing by the toy area and sending my nephew a movie of his favorite truck bin because he misses visiting us, which gives me an idea for a little children's story I can write and share on my Facebook Live, which reminds me I should defrost the Italian sausage for dinner.

6:00 p.m.: I'm now cooking dinner. In my workout clothes.

7:00 p.m.: I'm sitting at the table enjoying that dinner with a glass of wine, in my workout clothes.

8:00 p.m.: I give up and take a shower.

8:30 p.m.: I settle in with my twelve-year-old daughter and our beloved TV friends, *The Gilmore Girls*.

Halfway through five of Lorelai and Rory's seven glorious seasons, I'm reminded that Lorelai (the mom) has never burned a calorie or gone running in a single episode. She is too busy running her own business, while surviving on coffee and a truck driver's diet. My daughter Lucie and I have been joyfully bingeing the show throughout the quarantine era, watching Rory and Lorelai hit Luke's diner for pancakes every morning and crunch their way through a full bag of chips on their couch at night. We adore these crazy women who never exercise, and often treat ourselves to an extra episode on our own couch at night.

It's not that I don't want to work out. It's not that I don't have time. I have plenty of time.

"Should we watch one more, Mom?"

Sure, why not. We've got plenty of time.

🕐

Christina Geist is the author of Sorry Grown-Ups, You Can't Go to School. *She is also the founder of Boombox Gifts and co-founder of True Geist, a branding firm.*

The Retro Workout That Changed My Life

DYLAN LAUREN

How aqua jogging keeps me in balance.

I don't believe in deprivation, and I've never been successful with "all or nothing" diets.

As much as I love the taste of candy, I also love its vibrant colors, interesting textures, and the happiness that just looking at the stuff can evoke.

I taste test all the samples that come to our offices at Dylan's Candy Bar every day. For this reason—as well as many others—scheduling time to work out is crucial. I love exercising because it builds muscle and burns fat, but I also find that after a long day of work, exercise clears my head, reduces my stress level, and gives me a high that makes me feel accomplished. I love running long distances in the park, playing tennis, biking for miles on country roads, hiking, or hitting the gym if I can't get outside. (In fact, while writing this essay I'm typing on my BlackBerry while climbing on the StairMaster—the same way I wrote my book, *Dylan's Candy Bar: Unwrap Your Sweet Life!*)

I dislike sitting still for long periods of time; I prefer to multitask and keep moving. Having two athletic older brothers and a tomboy mother was probably key in shaping my active lifestyle. When I can't find the time to work out or if I'm injured, I feel crazed like an animal in a cage, almost overflowing with pent-up energy.

Injury has long been my worst enemy. When I was nine years old, I sprained my knee while waterskiing at camp and had to use crutches for nearly the entire summer. I was devastated to miss out on all of the fun sports like tennis, soccer, and volleyball. I was instructed to swim as much as possible to help rehab my leg and stay aerobically fit for when I recovered. As much as I didn't like the idea of swimming in the frigid and mysterious water of my camp's lake, I forced myself to do it because I had no other way to get exercise.

> I don't believe in deprivation and have never been successful at "all or nothing" diets.

Every day since, I am so glad I didn't quit.

Later, when I was in college at Duke, I got hurt again after running long distances without proper preparation. I had pulled my iliotibial band and had micro tears in my hamstring, so I took up swimming to help my recovery. One day at the pool, I came across a few Duke football and basketball players in the lane next to me. They were swimming, but also mixing it up by running in the swim lane, doing jumping jacks, treading water while playing catch, and doing some funny-looking dance moves.

I had witnessed eighty-year-olds in 1930s-style swim caps doing gentle water aerobics before, but seeing these muscular Duke athletes in action? That was a game changer for me.

For the next few weeks, I headed to the pool to study the athletes' movements. I created routines by incorporating their moves with my own, mimicking everything from spinning to recumbent biking, cross-country skiing, jumping rope, kickboxing, dancing, and sprints. After each session, I'd come out of the water completely exhausted and actually happier than I used to get after a long-distance run. I loved seeing the muscle tone I was developing everywhere and feeling the endorphin high without the pain of high-impact aerobics, and as much as I missed being outside in nature, being in the water cleared my head in the same way.

Friends and family members who at first thought I was crazy to go off and hang out in a freezing lake or random pool soon began to join me. In the past twenty years, I am proud to say I have turned many skeptics into aqua jogging converts. I've taught friends of all kinds to aqua jog; anyone bored with their regular gym routine or trying to avoid high-impact aerobics due to pregnancy or injury is a perfect candidate for aqua jogging. I've helped my parents save time and pain by curating customized low-impact aqua routines for them; on vacations, local lifeguards and hotel guests have joined me in the sea to try a new workout. Even my four-year-old twins, Kingsley Rainbow and Cooper Blue, have learned to feel comfortable in the water by mimicking some of Mommy's aqua moves!

> I had witnessed eighty-year-olds in 1930s-style swim caps doing gentle water aerobics before, but seeing these muscular Duke athletes in action? That was a game changer for me.

Aqua jogging has helped me balance my love of sweets and my work at the Candy Bar with my desire to stay fit, but I also love the built-in opportunity to multitask by being social and helping others while I work out. I of course never enjoyed being injured (who does?), but looking back, I'm able to appreciate the life lessons that came as a result of my injuries. I have turned to aqua jogging in the broiling hot summers, in the freezing winter, and when traveling for work; I simply find the nearest body of water—pool, ocean, lake, or lagoon—and I dive right in.

⊕

Dylan Lauren is the CEO and founder of Dylan's Candy Bar, the candy emporium and lifestyle brand. She is the author of Dylan's Candy Bar: Unwrap Your Sweet Life.

Breaking Up with My Kids

RACHEL LEVY LESSER

It's not them, it's me.

A few months ago, I was sitting on the cold, hard bleachers at my son's high school basketball game, when I found myself focused less on the game being played in front of me and more on the home team's bench. I was watching my son, who had been sitting there for a while. It seemed to me that he had spent a significantly larger portion of the game sitting on that bench than he had spent actually playing on the court.

He didn't look thrilled.

He looked kind of miserable.

I was looking for some sort of reassurance from my husband—that the coach would put our son back in the game soon and a smile would return to his face—when my aunt, who had come along with my uncle to watch the game, leaned in toward my left ear and said softly but firmly, "Sometimes you have to divorce yourself from kids—even for just a little while."

I nodded and looked back down toward the court, pretending to watch the game, which my son was not currently any part of, wondering what the hell my aunt was talking about.

Over the course of the past sixteen years, my aunt has become like a surrogate mother to me, having lost my own mom around the time my son was born. I trusted her wisdom. So, over coffee a couple of weeks later, I inquired about this divorcing yourself from your kids advice.

My aunt explained to me that as her kids got older—they are now fully grown with children of their own—she found she sometimes had to separate herself from them when they were going through a particularly tough time. I might want to do the same, she suggested, after witnessing me look more upset about my son not getting ample playing time than he did. This kind of distance would help both me and my kids, she explained.

> Sometimes you have to divorce yourself from kids—even for just a little while.

This advice was completely counterintuitive to me. When my kids were struggling with something, I would talk to them about what was going on, about what was bothering them, and then I'd offer suggestions. I wanted to help make things better in any and every way that I possibly could. This is my job, after all, and I pride myself on being pretty good at it.

Or so I thought.

This was, incidentally, the same aunt who had once described to me what being a mom felt like: She said it was like going out into the world every day, business as usual, except your own heart is off walking around somewhere else, outside of your body. That had made perfect sense to me. On the night of the game, my heart was a sad sixteen-year-old boy, sitting on the bench of a high school basketball court. My heart has also been, at times, a fourteen-year-old girl in a seemingly chronic bad mood, facing ever-fluctuating hormones.

It hurts to have my heart walking around outside of my body.

Perhaps, then, it was time for me to divorce my kids? I told my aunt I'd consider it. We could just take a little break (like Ross and

Rachel in *Friends*) and then we could get back together—just like everyone knew those characters inevitably would.

My breakup with my kids was hard, which shouldn't have come as such a shock to me; I'm not good at breakups! I've been in a relationship with the same hairdresser for more than twenty years. I'm still in the process of getting over a few ancient boyfriend breakups, and I can't even think about that one time I had to break up with a girlfriend.

One night, I forced myself to walk out of our family room, leaving my son to sulk alone on the couch in the dark after an especially long day. When my daughter launched into a laundry list of complaints about schoolwork another evening, I didn't take the bait. I told her it sounded like a lot, but I knew she could handle it—and that she had no choice but to handle it. Then, I went into the other room to do my own work. It was difficult to do but, surprisingly, my heart didn't hurt quite as much as I thought it would.

> The more they could see me not getting so upset, so involved, so invested in their problems and in things not always going their way, the more weight was lifted from their shoulders.

Eventually, I came to understand what my aunt meant about these little breakups being better for my kids, too. The more they could see me not getting so upset, so involved, so invested in their problems and in things not always going their way, the more weight was lifted from their shoulders. I actually remembered a few times in the past when they had tried to make me feel better about my worrying about them! I definitely didn't want to continue down that path.

So, I continue to divorce my kids every once in a while. I'm not even sure they're aware of it when we're on these breaks, but that's okay. I know it. And I know that it's good for all of us. I also know that we will inevitably get back together at some point, and we do. That's always my favorite part.

Rachel Levy Lesser is the author of Life's Accessories: A Memoir (and Fashion Guide) *and several other books.*

I Finally Learned to Dance Like Nobody's Watching

COURTNEY MAUM

**After birthing a child, my body
found new ways to move.**

My first attempt at public dance was at a surprise party for my thirteenth birthday. The event was a big deal: I went to an all-girls' school, and the party was a coed affair with imported boys. My mother took camcorder footage of me attempting to find "The Rhythm of the Night," and shifting into moroseness when nobody wanted to slow dance to "Nothing Compares to You." Watching the tape afterward, I zeroed in on my body—which had developed more quickly than my classmates'—bopping in a crowd of khaki pants and ponytails. I looked jumbly and uncomfortable. I was horrified.

Over the next few years, I braved a variety of athletic pursuits but dance wasn't one of them. My attempts at rhythmic movement lived and died within that fête. Though I certainly became more comfortable with my body as I aged, I had absolutely no desire to shake my frame around. In my teens and in my twenties, I felt discombobulated and ungainly, more gesundheit than gazelle.

It wasn't until I was pregnant that I got the hang of my own shape. I'd been doing yoga for years like a good girl from

Connecticut, and one day while in triangle pose my baby kicked me into an important realization: I did not like yoga. I was bored out of my skull with yoga. I suddenly realized that during this time of profound stillness and incubation, I wanted—and needed—to move the hell around.

In my second trimester, I put on big-beat music like Major Lazer and the French electronic artist Sophie, and I popped and locked and posed. After years of resenting my curves, I'd finally figured out what to do: I could drop it to the ground. I could drop it like it was hot. I got harder, faster, stronger to the music of Daft Punk.

Of the many gifts that motherhood can bring, one (for me, at least) was the cessation of caring what people thought about my body. All of my muscles and organs and bones had worked together to birth my daughter, and I wanted to celebrate our hard work. So I kept on dancing. I put on louder music and danced with my girl in her baby carrier all around the living room. When she developed sea legs, we hung a Jolly Jumper from the ceiling so that we could bounce together. The neighbors could see us waltzing from the window, the postman found me sweaty whenever he dropped a package off. But I wasn't embarrassed to move in public any longer—my mother body brought me joy. In addition to the mounting pride I felt, my actual structure got better after childbirth, too. My body grew longer and more supple, stretchy and more languorous, like a house finally settling into the ground on which it's built. Episiotomy be damned, I could touch my toes from a seated position. I could do a pirouette and land in fourth position; my daughter was my spot.

It wasn't until I was pregnant that I got the hang of my own shape.

My love affair with movement flourished as my child crawled from infancy to toddlerhood. I signed up for the community classes offered by Jacob's Pillow in the Berkshires, a seasonal opportunity that allows plebeians like me to join professional dancers in their morning warm-ups. There was only about ten minutes of chaste stretching before we were ordered to leap and fall and tumble (elegantly) across the ground. This exercise—which took place in front of actual professionals, mind you—would have been my idea of hell when I was younger, but something magnificent happened as I rolled across the freezing floor: because I didn't care if anyone was watching me, nobody did.

In my experiments with public dance classes, this lesson has been repeated for me on a larger scale. Being comfortable in your body is a gift, of course, but it's also a gift for others. When you spend time around people who actually like themselves, you can't help but be tempted to accept yourself more, too. In the years since Jacob's Pillow, I've tried everything on the menu in our Massachusetts corner: tango, belly dancing, hip hop, ballet, modern dance, online Masala Bhangra videos, even contra dance. When I'm on book tour, my Ballet Beautiful subscription is the first thing I pack, moving along to the founder's port de bras, attitudes, and demi plies via video in my hotel room. To the endless delight of my daughter, I'm the only parent who appears in the back of the little Zoom square during her online ballet classes. I figure if she's going to spend forty-five minutes sashaying around our bedroom, why can't I?

> Of the many gifts that motherhood can bring, one . . . was the cessation of caring what people thought about my body.

The weather has been bad in our Northeast corner during COVID-19: cold and gray and rainy, the kind of damp that makes you want to binge-watch *Ozark* instead of going for a walk. And so I turn to dance to shake my fear and sadness out. My husband joins us in our impromptu dance parties in the living room; we let our daughter jump from couch to couch. We can't travel, we can't plan, we can't go to the town lake. But inside of our houses, we're still called to move.

🕐

Courtney Maum is the author of multiple books including the novels Touch *and* Costalegre *and the nonfiction guide* Before *and* After the Book Deal.

Racing against the Coronavirus: How Working Out Is Keeping Me Sane

ZIBBY OWENS

I need to work out.

I'd been comfortably ignoring this truth while managing my four kids' logistical mayhem and building my business. But these uncertain and terrifying times have shown me how much I depend on it.

Emotionally. Physically.

Several weeks ago, as news of the coronavirus's inevitable arrival in the United States seeped into my consciousness, I started to panic. This wasn't a test. This wasn't a movie. It was coming. And I needed to plan. To protect my kids.

To take cover.

At first I was dealing with mundane things like rearranging plans for spring break and canceling flights. I quickly moved into preparing for all the kids' schools to be shut for months. Next thing I knew, hospitals up the street were considering building tents to prepare for the onslaught of patients. (I still can't believe this is currently in place.)

Was this actually happening? I thought that in this hyper-speed day and age, we were impervious to these types of horror-story afflictions.

Oh, how wrong I was.

As I raced around the apartment packing up the kids, shutting down my podcast, trying to find the birth certificates, my divorce agreement, all of our passports, my sentimental jewelry, I felt hysteria overtaking me. I was shaking. Quaking. Crying. Although even in my panic I knew how fortunate I was to be able to leave

I thought that in this hyper-speed day and age, we were impervious to these types of horror-story afflictions.

New York City when others couldn't.

That age-old fight-or-flight instinct took hold: I had to run.

Right then.

Urgently.

As a recreational jogger once or twice a month, I found this intense urge curious and unexpected.

But I listened to my body. I stopped packing, changed into my workout clothes—which, if I'm being honest, had gotten a little tight—and descended down into my building's basement gym.

A typical "workout" for me involved reading on the elliptical machine for thirty minutes, barely breaking a sweat. This time, I blasted music in my headphones, cranked up the speed on the treadmill and sprinted. My legs spun, my arms pumped, and I zoomed. (Back when "zoom" meant to go fast, not to communicate with the outside world.)

The music blaring was equally therapeutic. The lyrics took on new meaning, like in Jess Glynne's "Hold My Hand": "Tryna find a moment where I can find release."

The kids' *Frozen 2* soundtrack seemed wise and prophetic, especially the song, "Into the Unknown": "Every day's a little harder as I feel your power grow."

That first day I only ran for seventeen minutes until my older daughter came down to the gym asking me to help her find her homework. But it was enough. My face was almost purple with exertion, my heart was pumping, and I felt suddenly free. Uplifted. Empowered.

I did it again the next day. And the next. Until the car groaned under our heavy load and we headed out of town to hide out for the foreseeable future.

I've kept up the running. Even just twenty minutes a day is enough for me to emotionally reset, to find a slice of calm in the chaos, to re-center me so I can parent more effectively. I've gone running outside on the squishy grass as the last drops of rain splattered down. I've done online workout videos with the kids, dancing to Kidz Bop.

Every day, a little something.

This time is simply terrifying. My natural inclination to plan has been thwarted. I can't see past this day, this hour. If I peer out at what's coming, I panic. Will I get sick? Will my parents be okay? What about everyone else I love and care about? How will everyone in the country be able to eat and pay the rent if no businesses are open and no services can be provided? What will happen as a result of millions of people essentially being imprisoned in their own homes with no release date in sight?

I don't know the answers to these questions.

I can't know.

All I can do is keep my head down, try to find meaning in the world by helping others, particularly those in the literary community, and pray. One hour at a time.

Moving my body is keeping me sane. So I'll keep squeezing into my sports bra and lacing up my sneakers as we all weather this storm together.

Minute by minute. Mile by mile.
Into the unknown.

Zibby Owens is a writer and mother of four in New York City. She is a literary advocate and the creator and host of the award-winning literary podcast Moms Don't Have Time to Read Books. *She runs a literary salon with author events, a virtual book club, and a daily Z-IGTV live author interview series.*

How a Failed Relationship Made Me a Runner

JILL SANTOPOLO

My ex taught me how to run.

Well, that's not entirely true. I learned how to run when I was a kid, sprinting—down the field in soccer games or racing a few quick steps before turning a round-off into a back-handspring in gymnastics. But he taught me how to be a runner. He taught me endurance, how to race, and what it means to keep going when you think your body is ready to give out.

We started dating in February, and it didn't take long for me to realize that he was an exercise guy. He had a gym membership and ran miles and miles in Central Park, even though it was cold outside. My own exercise consisted solely of walking to and from work. The walk took about half an hour each way, and it was one of my favorite parts of the day. I would pop in my earbuds and zone out, letting my mind wander, thinking about everything and nothing at all.

Winter became spring, and he tore a tendon in his ankle and had to undergo surgery. As soon as he was able, he was back in Central Park, first walking, and then back to running once again. He told me it was easier for him to think when he ran. I had since gotten a new job, one that required taking a forty-minute subway ride in each direction. I thought about my walks back and forth to work, and I wondered if running would feel like that—like my mind could get lost in itself.

So, that fall, I told him I wanted to run, too, and asked if he would teach me how. On our first run together, he told me to go at whatever pace I wanted, and he would match it, and we'd see how long I could manage. We jogged together in the park, me breathing hard—him, not so much—for about fifteen minutes. At that point, we'd gone from West 72nd Street down the bottom loop and back up, almost to 72nd Street on the East Side. I told him I needed to stop, and he pointed to East 72nd Street, about half a block away.

I found that I loved not only running, but also racing. It gave my mind a chance to unfurl, and it felt good to push my body to become stronger and faster.

"You can make it to there," he said. "Then we'll stop."

I didn't think I could, but I did. And then we walked home. That was lesson one.

We got into a groove on the weekends. We'd start out running together, I'd go as far as I could—and then a little more—and after that, I'd head home and he'd finish his run. He encouraged me to register for races, some of which we did together and some of which I did on my own, with him cheering me on. He taught me to push hard up a hill, to always run on the outside of the pack at the beginning of a race, and not to drink every cup of water that was offered. With his tips, I found that I loved not only running, but also racing. It gave my mind a chance to unfurl, and it felt good to push my body to become stronger and faster.

The following spring, I decided to train for a half marathon, and he helped me make a plan. I'd never felt stronger in my life. At the finish line, he seemed just as proud as I was.

But, like that race, our relationship finished, too. I lost him, but I didn't lose running. One weekend, as I was running in the park, I saw someone wearing a triathlon shirt. I'm going to do that, I decided. I wasn't a swimmer, and I hadn't ridden a bike in a while, but I hadn't been a runner either. I knew it would take time and work. But I had time and I wasn't afraid of work.

I went online and found a sprint triathlon that was taking place at the end of July. That gave me sixteen weeks. I found a sixteen-week schedule I could follow, and then signed up. My first day in the pool was miserable. My first day on a bike was only marginally better. But I kept at it.

As the summer progressed, I visited my parents at their beach house, and my dad—a former collegiate athlete himself—decided he was going to be my coach. He stood at the ocean's edge timing my laps in the buoyed-off area of the beach. I told him that time wasn't important to me—I just wanted to reach the finish line.

The day of the race arrived, and I was ready. My parents came to cheer me on. When we got there, I found out that there was a serious undertow happening in the Atlantic Ocean. I didn't let it worry me until I got in and realized how hard I had to tread water in order to keep myself from floating backward.

That swim was one of the most difficult things I have ever done—physically and emotionally. Halfway through, I thought I would have to give up; I wasn't strong enough to overpower the undertow. But one of the lifeguards on a paddle-board told me to float for a while, and then get back to it. I thought

But like that race, our relationship finished, too. I lost him, but I didn't lose running.

of the way I would always push myself just a little further than I thought I could when I was learning to run. I flipped back over, and I swam.

The bike portion of the race came as a welcome relief after finally making it out of the water, and then, last was the run. I was pretty far toward the back of the pack when I started, but as soon as my sneakers hit the asphalt, I felt a surge of strength. My mind focused, and I felt the familiar rhythm of my footfalls. I pushed hard up the hill, and I crossed the finish line. I made it.

As I took a bottle of lemon-flavored sports drink from the table, I thought about how every experience we have shapes who we are. There's no way I would have completed that race if my past had been any different. And in that moment, I was grateful. Grateful that a failed relationship had made me a runner.

🕐

Jill Santopolo is the internationally bestselling author of novels The Light We Lost *and* More Than Words.

These Days, I'm Running to Stay Sane

SARA SHEPARD

I put on shoes and slide headphones in my ears. If it's cold, I add a hat, sometimes with a pompom on it, which bobs as I move, reminding me that it's still there. My gloves are sometimes high-tech ones from New Balance but are just as often woolen mittens from Anthropologie or gloves so old the fingertips are fraying away.

I'm not the runner who's in fashion or whose clothes even remotely match. I sweat a lot, and my skin gets unattractively red, and I'm not in neon-colored trendy sneakers but utilitarian black men's shoes that are an update of an update of an update of a running shoe I was specifically measured for at a Super Runner's Shop on 24th Street and 3rd Avenue in New York City in 1997. I have been wearing the same brand and make of sneakers, more or less, for twenty-three years.

That's how long I've been a runner. Longer than that, actually. And every day, regardless of the weather, I go outside and do the same thing. I run the same neighborhoods, by the same houses. Often, I see the same people, or the same people see me.

"Oh, I saw you running," they'll tell me later. "You're really dedicated. Are you training for something?"

No, I tell them. I'm almost never training for anything. For better or worse, this is just what I do.

When I was a kid, running was a means to flirt with boys on the junior high track team. In high school, it became an obsession and bridge to disordered eating. For a while, running was my favorite mode of punishment, a symptom of what I now understand was and is an illness. After moving to New York City, I slowly recovered. I regained a healthy balance. Since then, running has become a helpful aid in the writing process—I've been cracking big plot points mid-run for a good fifteen years now. The minutes of breathlessness serve as a time where I can work out complicated feelings.

While all those parts of my history with running are true, the sport has taken on a whole new meaning in the face of the coronavirus pandemic. Now, every time I step outside—and let me be clear, my running path keeps a safe distance from people—it isn't just my workout for the day. It's a valuable, life-saving routine. It's a meditation. It's an escape.

This isn't my first time running through big, scary moments in history. Post 9/11, I ran around Prospect Park in Brooklyn—the air still smelled like charred electronics and death—and tried to cope. When the banks crashed in 2008, I was living in Tucson, Arizona, and my house was abruptly valued at a hundred thousand dollars less than what I'd bought it at, and I ran on back trails amid rattlesnakes and coyotes and tried to figure out what to do. In 2012, I went through a difficult separation and divorce not long after having my first child, and I ran on a tranquil, wooded trail to try to dull my pain. Running has been a constant no matter what happened; often, when I return from a run, I feel better, more centered, calm.

> For a while, running was my favorite mode of punishment, a symptom of what I now understand was and is an illness.

And now, in the face of COVID-19, it's no different. On some of my latest runs, my mind keeps churning over the same brutal questions: When is this going to end? How can we stay safe? Is my career secure? What if my parents get this illness?

But there's also one big difference between running amid those other crises and running through this one: I have children. Thinking, questioning, needy children—who, as it turns out, are now out of school for the rest of the year. So it's not just my struggles I'm working out when I'm running these days—it's also theirs.

Like so many people, I'm trying to work from home with my kids now home as well. We're limping along. At almost six and eight, they have somewhat of a grasp of what's going on—though certainly not the unprecedented nature of it all—and at the moment, they're chill about staying home from school. They've Skyped with friends and teachers. They've played outside. We've gone for (safe, socially distant) walks. But they've also watched a lot of YouTube, played tons of video games and Minecraft, and made ridiculous TikTok videos. On their first day off, I kept to a schedule of reading, math, science, and spelling. But as the week progressed and the news got grimmer and more real, that all went to hell. I wanted to say, oh it's okay—it's only been a week.

> Every person in the world shouldn't be consumed with the same thoughts and worries all at the same time. It just doesn't seem right, and yet here it is.

Now I've lost track of what week we're on.

On my runs now, I'm not breaking any speed records or even pushing myself very hard. I'm barely listening to audiobooks (I keep having to rewind the thriller I've been listening to over and over because I can't stay on top of the plot) and I'm shying away from every podcast in my feed, and I'm having trouble even brainstorming new books to write. Instead, I go out and run my miles and try as best I can to tamp down my anxiety. I think through worst-case scenarios. I make plans. I make lists. I allow myself to be distracted and scared and frazzled and irrational while I'm on the road, running alone, and after an hour passes, the feelings aren't necessarily out of my system—they come back in the middle of the night, and keep me awake for hours. (Is anyone sleeping well amid this?) But that solid block of time of movement plus intense worry plus sweat plus the outdoors works. I come home a little more peaceful and centered.

I am lucky. I know this. I am lucky because I have a good immune system, and because I have an emergency fund (though, like many others, it has dwindled), and because everyone I know at the moment is safe. I'm also lucky because I can still run—physically, yes, but also because my running path is appropriately socially distant. I feel for those living in New York or other busy cities where running while staying safe might not be as possible. I feel for people whose lifeline was, say, the elliptical machine at the gym and don't have a comparable machine at home.

Now, every time I step outside—and let me be clear, my running path keeps a safe distance from people—it isn't just my workout for the day. It's a valuable, life-saving routine. It's a meditation. It's an escape.

But mostly, I just feel for all of us right now. Whenever a person pops in my head—someone from my past, an ex-boyfriend, a random celebrity—I think, Good Lord, they're dealing with this, too. It's a bizarre feeling, and though it's one of connectedness, it's a connectedness of the worst kind. The whole world is suffering. For me, trying to conceptualize this is akin to staring into the sky at night and trying to grasp that the universe is infinite: it seems impossible. Every person in the world shouldn't be consumed with the same thoughts and worries all at the same time. It just doesn't seem right, and yet here it is.

So I'm going to say what a lot of people have already said, but bears repeating: get through this as best you can. Do what you need to do. If it's that an extra glass of wine every night, go for it. If it's eating extra carbs and watching terrible TV—thank God, there's still TV—huzzah. And if you're like me, maybe it's lacing up your shoes and going for a run even though it's pouring rain. We just have to get through this.

And we will.

🕐

Sara Shepard is the #1 bestselling author of the Pretty Little Liars *series and many other books, including her most recent novel,* Reputation.

What Locker-Room Talk Sounds Like to Me

BONNIE TSUI

When indoor pools closed, I missed my community in the changing room the most.

There are so many things to miss in this pandemic time. In summer—the season of the swimmer—family reunions, camps, and vacations are largely absent. The things we rely upon for mental and physical health are no longer readily available. Lately, I've been missing my community pool, where the locker room was a tableau on aging. There were bodies and bottoms of every sort on display, from squishy baby to saggy lady. But it was not the kind of place where short-lived resolutions to lose fifteen pounds got made or broken. The arc of fitness was long there, and it bent toward seniors.

Pre-pandemic, the hour in which I frequented the pool for my laps coincided with the 8 a.m. aqua aerobics class, taught by Kathe, a calm, convivial woman with honey-colored hair and a beatific smile. Many of her devotees ranged into their eighties. Some were there for physical therapy after an injury; others were contending with the incessant aches and pains of age. In that damp little maze of shared benches and open showers, where every flick of a towel or reach of an arm brought you into someone else's personal space, ordinary civilities carried larger import.

I am not eighty. But among those eighty-year-olds is where I liked to be.

I first came to this pool after my second child was born and my family moved across the bay from San Francisco to Berkeley. It's where I reclaimed my body, a little softer and a lot more tired, as my own. Day after day in the outdoor pool, I pulled and kicked my way back into the swimming habits that made me feel like, well, me. More than five years later, my passage through each day was eased by the morning transit through this locker room, in the company of these women. The daily celebration of bodies that are happy and working made me comfortable and ever grateful in mine.

I am not eighty. But among those eighty-year-olds is where I liked to be.

As a lifelong swimmer, I've found that my morning workouts smoothed away the edges, both strengthening and calming my restless body, so I could face the world with equanimity. But as I got older, I found that the locker room itself did something different for me.

It was where we warmed up from the swim in the communal showers; where we jockeyed for space in the crowded dressing area, all of us in various stages of nakedness: this one applying moisturizer, that one in underwear, still another wrestling with a stubborn pair of leggings. We contorted our bodies in the most unattractive ways. It was where we showed vulnerability, in all its forms, and felt safe doing it.

Loneliness, we know, deteriorates health. I listened to the way the people in this room rallied around each other—through struggles that ranged from family discord and sleeping woes to cancer and chemo and the death of dear friends. Sometimes I swam with a buddy, or trained with the Masters team. Often I came alone. But I always found company in the locker room—a conversation to dip into, or just to overhear. And there was always the comforting routine of simply discussing the water conditions in the pool that day, or admiring the pattern on someone else's bathing suit.

Certainly there were maternal and grand-maternal surrogates to be found there. Once, as we were getting dressed, I confessed to a friend that I didn't know how to buy underwear anymore because all of it comes from my mother. She could eyeball the ideal fit of a bikini brief for me from a mile away and she refreshed my collection of undergarments every year in my Christmas stocking without fail. Another woman, perhaps a decade older than we were, listened to the story and got teary.

> I listened to the way the people in this room rallied around each other—through struggles that ranged from family discord and sleeping woes to cancer and chemo and the death of dear friends.

"That is the sweetest thing I ever heard," she said, wiping her eyes. "You should tell your mom I said so." And so I did.

There was also wisdom and kinship on tap. Kathe dispensed nuggets about everything from mah-jong and yoga classes to the history of Title IX at nearby UC Berkeley, where she was once a student. Alicia showed Patricia her longtime stretching routine by getting right down atop her towel on the clammy tiled floor.

"I have been stretching all my life; I have scoliosis," Alicia declared, mid-hip stretch. "If I didn't do it, I'd be in a wheelchair now."

Lovely Patricia with her British accent chirped anxiously above her, "I'm glad you're not! But I think you'd better get up now dear, or you'll get run over!"

As they sailed or shuffled or sauntered out of the locker room, the ladies called to everyone to have a lovely day. When they passed me at the long mirror by the door, they smiled and met my eyes, making me feel there was a solution for most every problem.

Locker room talk? This was our kind of locker room talk:

How are you?

I'm OK. I'm here, aren't I?

The cackling laughter leaked out into the hallway. I could hear it all the way from the pool deck.

These days, three thousand miles away from a mother and grandmother and a gaggle of aunts I don't know when I'll see next, I think often of that laughter, and find a small measure of comfort in anticipating opening day at the pool.

🕐

Bonnie Tsui is a journalist and the author of Why We Swim.

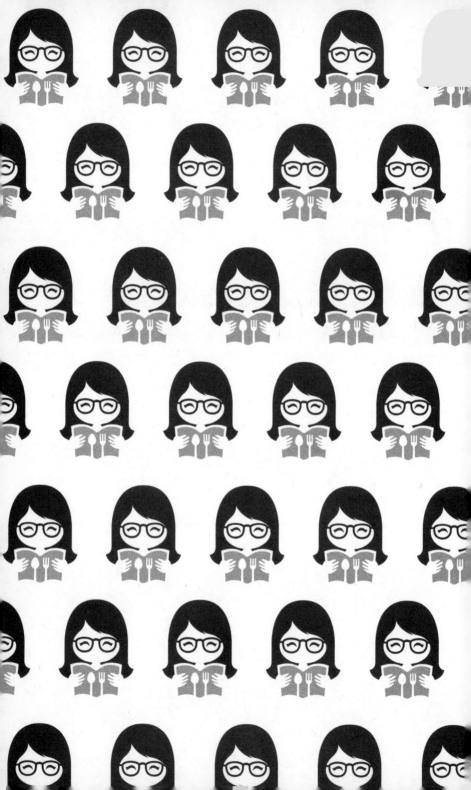

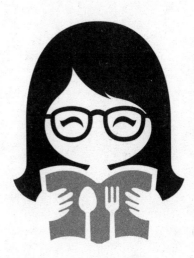

MOMS
DON'T HAVE
TIME TO
EAT

My Mother Says No
ELISSA ALTMAN

At first, the deliveries were small and biweekly. A roast chicken and braised flanken from her favorite local kosher restaurant, which, after eighty years in business, shuttered in the early days of the virus, perhaps presaging end times. Then came the comfort food orders that I was able to phone in from my home in Connecticut: chicken potpie, lasagna, quiche. All freezable. And then, finally, there were the dishes I delivered to her when the basic food items upon which she depends—bread, eggs—started to become scarce in Manhattan: quarts of homemade chicken soup that I made late into a weeknight, waking the following morning at six to skim the fat from its surface, ladling it, bleary-eyed, into freezable containers; minestrone; sautéed broccoli with confited garlic that she could pick at in the middle of the night or fold together with some egg whites because, as she likes to remind me, yolks are fattening.

The next day, I walked into my mother's Manhattan apartment with a restaurant-grade, heavy-duty insulated bag, plunked it down on her counter, unzipped it, and opened her freezer door to begin stocking it. There was no room: at one hundred pounds, she had eaten almost nothing I'd sent her in weeks, although she assured me she had.

I wasn't hungry, she said, shrugging. Do you want me to be big and fat? I'll never be a star.

She looked me up and down. She patted my stomach.

Also, she said, staring at my head, you need your color done.

My heart began to pound. I could feel the heat rise in waves off my face.

In middle age and at the suggestion of my cardiologist, I had recently restarted a long-abandoned meditation practice. I shelved my beloved red wine—I have what they used to call a hollow leg, according to my late father—and instead attempted self-care, after navigating life as the only child of this stunning, narcissistic personality disordered mother, a former television singer and an anorexic who didn't know she was pregnant with me for six months, and with whom I have such a codependent relationship that she often calls me fourteen times a day. A mother who said, when I went to cooking school in the late eighties, that I was doing it for spite because, as she put it, food is the enemy.

> There would be peace and beauty amid the dark unknown.

So I took a breath. I eyed the box of spigot Pinot Grigio I'd left in her fridge a few weeks earlier.

If this gets bad, I said to her, I'm going to have to come get you and bring you back to Connecticut for a while.

No, she said. *I will not* come.

You'll have to—you're eighty-four. You're high risk.

Are you calling me old? How *dare* you.

I zipped up my insulated bag. I kissed her on the cheek. And I left.

For the next two weeks, my wife of twenty years—we call her Saint Susan—and I begged my mother to let us bring her to our house in the country, where we could care for her and keep her safe. And, of course, feed her.

No, she said, her television blaring in the background. I'm watching *Play Misty for Me*. It's my favorite.

I could hear the bloodcurdling screams seventy-five miles away.

I want to make sure you're eating, I pleaded. You need to stay strong, Ma.

I'm eating fine, she said. Did you get your color done?

Every day for two weeks, her answer was the same: No.

Until it wasn't.

When can you get me, she asked one morning. I'm starting to get nervous.

Susan and I filled our refrigerators and freezer with the things that would keep us all healthy and fed: soups and stews, sourdough breads, whole chickens, pork roasts. Trained years ago in the art of restaurant repurposing, I could take care of us and feed us well for a few months. We would be okay. And then I drove into the city to pick up my mother and bring her home. Our little family would be together, under one roof, hunkered down. We would heal. There would be peace and beauty amid the dark unknown.

These are uncertain times, and we have taken in this most difficult, complicated woman whose relationship with me sits at the traumatic core of my life.

Our first dinner together was roast chicken and a salad.

My mother pushed the food around on her plate, making small piles here and there, and then fed bits of chicken to Petey, our dog.

You need to buy a stationary bicycle like the one I have, she said, out of the blue.

To keep the weight off.

And then she went to bed.

In the days that have followed, my mother has taken in roughly six hundred daily calories, most in the form of the miniature cupcakes that she picks at in the night when Susan and I are asleep. I called her doctor in New York for advice.

How do I feed her? I asked.

She's a miracle of modern science, the doctor said. Also, there is nothing you can do. You and your wife need to stay safe. Stay alive. And remember your blood pressure.

Twenty years ago, I fled Manhattan for New England; after a lifetime of acrimony and blame and the toxic knot of the maternal gone awry, I broke up with my mother because, a as a physician once told me, my health was on the line. I have not lived under the same roof with her since Reagan was in office. But these are uncertain times, and as Susan and I promised each other we would long before coronavirus was part of our lexicon, we have taken in this most difficult, complicated woman whose relationship with me sits at the traumatic core of my life, like the blazing sun.

We have to find a way to make it work, for however long.

There is one thing you can do, my mother's doctor said, when I called.

I waited for her wisdom.

Feed her more cupcakes.

⊕

Elissa Altman is the critically acclaimed author of Motherland: A Memoir of Love, Loathing and Longing, Treyf: My Life as an Unorthodox Outlaw, *and* Poor Man's Feast: A Love Story of Comfort, Desire, and the Art of Simple Cooking.

In Russia, Luggage Lost, Identity Found

NINA RENATA ARON

Without my clothes and belongings, I discovered a new version of myself.

In my mid-twenties, I traveled to St. Petersburg, Russia, for the better part of a summer to immerse myself in the language before starting a PhD program. I wrote nervously in my journal on the trip from New York City as the flight attendants, pretty blondes clad in baby blue, walked the aisles serving drinks. Though I arrived safely, my luggage did not. To the dormitory where I was staying—a mammoth cement block—I rode the metro unencumbered, carrying only my purse and its assortment of essentials: my wallet, a book, gum, lip gloss, headphones.

"The suitcase will be at your building," an airport employee had told me roughly when I reported the missing bag, without even looking up, let alone looking up my name, address, or flight number. I almost laughed.

The suitcase never came, and for weeks, I couldn't get comfortable. At first, nightly, I washed the clothing I'd flown in—unflattering jeans, a baggy black T-shirt, and clogs—in the tiny bathroom sink. I got to know some of the women in the dorm, and borrowed a couple of things, but they didn't fit. I spent hours on the phone with the airline trying to track down the missing piece of luggage, as did my then-boyfriend in New York, but to no avail. Without my clothes, shoes, hair dryer, or beauty products, I didn't feel like myself. But I was too broke to shop. So I wore the same outfit every day. On the long, breezy escalator ride down into the metro station, I locked eyes with passing commuters on their way up. Who do they think I am? I wondered, with the narcissism of youth. They can't possibly tell anything about me.

Of course, I was not quite myself. Or I didn't know yet just who I was, who I wanted to be. Hadn't an element of self-discovery been baked into the trip itself? This was before marriage, motherhood, or divorce. I was a young woman, nondescript, alone in a dizzyingly foreign pastel city where the buildings looked like iced pastries and the sun never set. St. Petersburg is close to the Arctic Circle, so for a couple months a year the city dwells in the perpetual pinky twilight of White Nights. At night, I sat on a bench in a small park and read by the baffling natural light of 10:00 pm or 11:00 pm. During the day, after classes, I walked the city and visited literary museums dedicated to the writers I loved most: Akhmatova, Dostoevsky, Brodsky, Nabokov. I practiced the Russian language in front of a mirror, as I'd been told to, trying to let my mouth go slack enough to sound natural. Vodka helped. My accent improved, but still sounded faintly foreign. Where are you from? Russians asked. Chechnya? Georgia?

As the days passed, I forgot about the things I'd intended to bring with me to distinguish myself as American, or alluring. As an individual. I forgot about the winged black eyeliner I applied every day at home, the lipstick colors I considered my signature. Those were in a cloth bag, tucked between a layer of tank tops and a stack of floral skirts in a suitcase, somewhere in the world. I couldn't identify myself as cool with band shirts or my motorcycle jacket. I stopped trying to read others' reactions to me and started to pay closer attention to the city, to people.

Eventually I befriended Anya, a vivacious middle-aged Georgian woman who lived in an old train car at Moskovsky station. We met while browsing books. A couple nights a week, I brought her wine and brandy and she cooked me dinner. We made each other laugh, especially as I struggled to keep up with her rapid-fire questions about my life in New York. Hearing the story of my lost suitcase, Anya clasped her hands together, wincing and laughing, saying, "How terrible!" and really leaning into the word "terrible" for effect, as Russians often do. She began to loan me some of her own clothes, flamboyant, flowing, and diaphanous garments she thought were elegant but which were unlike anything I would ever have worn at home.

"Stylish!" she exclaimed, as I tried them on.

I started to say perhaps this wasn't really my style and then thought better of it. Anya gave me makeup too, including eyeshadow in that saturated late-Soviet blue color, which I decided—what the hell?—to wear when I went out in the evenings. It had been a month since I'd been legible as the self I knew back home, so I stopped trying. I leaned in to my discomfort and let my usual performance of myself unravel and become something different. By the time a new friend took me on a date to the opera at the end of my trip, I was speaking and feeling more Russian than I'd ever thought possible. And I was wearing one of Anya's dresses, a semi-sheer number, cinched at the waist, in a bold, swirling black-and-white print. The lipstick was hers, too: metallic and cotton-candy pink.

As the days passed, I forgot about the things I'd intended to bring with me to distinguish myself as American, or alluring.

Travel always has this effect, to some extent. It makes "the strange familiar and the familiar strange," in the spirit of anthropologist

Horace Miner. (I would learn that line later that year, in my graduate program). On this trip, without the usual markers of identity that kept me tethered to my sense of myself, the change to the texture of daily life was even starker, and ultimately more meaningful. I found a new freedom without those markers. I saw differently, noticed differently, and allowed myself to look out rather than constantly anticipating and managing being looked at.

It also felt like the universe might have designed the entire experience as a test. About two weeks after I returned to Brooklyn, my suitcase showed up on my doorstep. I didn't know where on earth it had been, but everything inside was intact and folded nicely, just as I'd packed it.

🕐

Nina Renata Aron is a journalist and the author of the debut memoir Good Morning, Destroyer of Men's Souls.

Hey, Food Network Addicts: This Is Our Time to Shine

DIBS BAER

What Guy, Giada, and Ina taught me about living in the moment.

Confession: I'm one of those annoying people on social media who posts pictures of all the food they're making. I've shared photos of blueberry scones, grilled cheese, my grandma's chicken soup, cake, cookies, pasta, sausages, even an ugly-AF egg salad sandwich. Oddly, I have not made the ubiquitous loaf of fresh-baked bread yet, although I'm hoarding plenty of yeast in my cupboard.

Don't tell anyone.

I'm so invested in my new hobby that I even started a Facebook group called "The Self-Quarantine 15" (har har), though many people are saying that it should really be nineteen because . . . well, you get it.

Just where did I get the (matzo) balls to post all of my ambitious yet mediocre offerings? Well, I've been training for this moment for a decade—actually since the first time I laid eyes on the Food Network. Like so many other home cooks addicted to Guy, Bree, Giada, Ina, and all the others, the pandemic forced me to step up and put my prolific television watching to good use. Like Nuke LaLoosh in *Bull Durham*, I was finally being called up to The Show. My family needed me to cook ASAP—and a lot.

Luckily, I'd logged ten thousand hours of intensive study. I was ready.

If you would've told me ten years ago that I'd be obsessed with cooking during a global pandemic, I would have laughed (and then cried. WTF is happening?!?). Chef Dibs was never really in the cards. I lived in Brooklyn for fifteen years, had the stereotypical busy New York City lifestyle, and probably made myself a proper meal . . . oh, I'm gonna say . . . five times?

It wasn't until eight years ago, when I moved to California, that I started to cook and bake, which I attribute to the fact that I finally had a real kitchen and a damn dishwasher. (From now on, I don't care if I live in a toolshed. My home will have a dishwasher.) Suddenly, I could experiment and make a mess with a ton of pots and pans. I baked breakfast casseroles, pulled pork in the slow cooker, and made Mario Batali's shrimp scampi. I tried to make things from scratch that you just assumed you couldn't, like bagels and Ding Dongs, because why not? I even put a grill on my patio—outdoor space!—and became a barbecue master (in my own mind).

Around this time, I started watching Food Network twenty-four/seven. And today, I think it's safe to say I've seen every episode of *Beat Bobby Flay* and the entire *Diners, Drive-Ins and Dives* series forty times. I'm not complaining. Alex and Sunny and Valerie, and even that Sandwich King guy, have become my cooking mentors. You can't watch that much Food Network and not learn how to cook even a little by osmosis.

If you would've told me ten years ago that I'd be obsessed with cooking during a global pandemic, I would have laughed (and then cried. WTF is happening?!?).

Their happy, hungry voices invade your brain and seep into your consciousness. My meditation mantra is now "All my recipes have to be approved by cowboys, hungry kids, and me!" And I don't even know any cowboys or have any kids.

All of this Food Network watching prepared me for two life-changing events.

First, five years ago, my dad passed away and I decided to move in with my mom in her Palm Springs retirement community. We needed each other and it just made sense. And that's when my cooking went to eleven—in terms of frequency, not skill.

When COVID-19 shut down basically everything, cooking for my mom and myself morning, noon, and night wasn't intimidating: it was my calling.

Due to a number of factors—including efficiency and my being "bossy," as my mom called it—I became the grocery shopper and main cook in our new household.

Also, my mom didn't like herbs. That's literally what she told me one day: "I don't like herbs." That was, um, limiting, given my new cooking prowess. So, to have more control over what I'd be eating, I staged a kitchen coup.

My mom didn't mind . . . too much. We both loved Food Network and had it on all day, so we'd see a dish on our favorite shows and give it a go, like Bacon Cheddar Twists with Soft Boiled Eggs from *Brunch at Bobby's* or a peach crumble by *The Pioneer Woman*. I made sure to make things I knew my mom loved, like shrimp and grits or eggs Benedict, though it took me way too many times to be able to not only poach an egg but get it out of the water intact.

My mom's a tough customer, so when she liked something, like my blender hollandaise sauce, she'd announce it was an "A+." She also told me repeatedly, "You make the best grilled cheese in the world," and I beamed every time, even though it's not that hard. (Room temperature butter, people!)

We also cooked together. Even though I'm more a savory fan and my mom has the sweet tooth, baking bonded us: I absolutely loved baking with my mom. It felt like we were mad scientists whipping up magic potions. Neither of us had any idea what baking powder or baking soda actually did, but we loved mixing all these random things into a bowl and . . . poof!, an hour later we were eating cake. How? Why? Didn't matter. It was all about the journey.

Nothing could prepare any of us for the second life-changing event—the devastating global pandemic we're in right now. But in terms of cooking? Who knew all that television watching would pay off? Because of my continuing education at Food Network and the fact that I was already cooking a ton, I was able to easily go from armchair chef to first string. When COVID-19 shut down basically everything, cooking for my mom and me morning, noon, and night wasn't intimidating: it was my calling.

As I write this, we are still trying new, often complicated recipes, because we have endless amounts of time to do so. I make mistakes—big mistakes—like the other night I messed up Trisha Yearwood's potato gnocchi so badly I actually spat it out and popped a frozen pizza in the oven.

But I will always cherish these memories of cooking with my mom. Of course, I cannot wait to get back to normal and have our world be safe and healthy again. I cannot wait to hang up my apron and let real culinary experts make outstanding food again for me in their wonderful restaurants.

And if that means Chef Dibs is sent back down to the minors, so be it. I'll happily take the demotion.

🕒

Dibs Baer is a New York Times *bestselling author. Her most recent book is* Lady Tigers in the Concrete Jungle: How Softball and Sisterhood Saved Lives in the South Bronx.

What the Brady Bunch Taught Me about Family Dinners

ALISON CAYNE

Like many little girls of the 1970s, my first true loves came in this order: my Barbie Dream House, my Easy-Bake Oven, and *The Brady Bunch*. I don't mean I liked just Bobby or Greg. I was fully into Alice, all the girls (not so much Marcia), the parents, and their floppy dog, Tiger. I watched *The Brady Bunch* the way some kids would eat a bowl of ice cream—I eagerly anticipated the next episode, inhaled it in rapture, and felt this hollow, homesick feeling when I knew the episode was coming to an end. The Bradys showed me how I wanted to live my life. I wanted braces. I wanted to carry my books in between my folded arms. I wanted car washes and cheerleading and family adventures. Mostly though, I wanted big family dinners around an abundant, boisterous table.

I was an only child, and a pretty lonely one at that. I have plenty of friends who loved being the only child in their family, reportedly totally satisfied with their own company and imaginations. Most of them opted to have "onlys" themselves, and still relish their time alone with their own thoughts. That was not and definitely is not the case for me. The moment the opportunity arose, I promptly had five children and built a business centered around home cooking. I even (inadvertently) found the Mike to my Carol: my new fiancé has two of his own children. We are a modern-day Brady Bunch. (We hear this a lot.) Big, floppy dog included.

For the most part, I have constructed the life the Bradys taught me to want. All of my life has been laser focused on creating abundant, boisterous tables, and for that I am extremely grateful. I taught myself to cook at eight years old. I started hosting dinner parties in middle school. I once made potato salad for two hundred people in the basement of a college dorm. When I had children,

Our family table has been the gossamer that has carried my family and me through illness, divorce, and now, a global pandemic.

I could finally cook for an army daily and shout, "Dinner!" like Carol would. It was the hallmark of my Hallmark family.

But there was a hitch. My model family—and this is quite obvious to me now—was not only fictional, but it set me up for a total misunderstanding of family life, how to be a mother, what sibling interaction looks like, and how "blended families" function. (Hint: the very name is a fallacy.) Every fight my kids had for the first decade (and let's face it, even now, dipping into my third decade of parenting) upset me. Not just because conflict makes me uncomfortable, but because it looked nothing like a Brady fight. Every dinner that ended in people storming off or plates left full, every flipped-over board game, every slammed door, all of it appeared in a split screen across my brain of Carol Brady and me. On Carol's side: understanding, resolution, and laughter. Across my half of the screen? A big stamp of failure and hopelessness. Carol Brady never blamed herself for Marcia's self-centeredness or Jan's deep insecurity. She never, in all five seasons, had a breakdown. Not once.

While *The Brady Bunch* created a completely unattainable standard, it also gave me a panacea in family dinners. Regardless of what is happening to or within my family, despite the steely silence or open hostility, we still sit down to dinner together every night. That's the rule. Some nights, dinner lasts three minutes before devolving; many nights we host people passing through town, or friends of friends. Most evenings we eat food that I've made, but sometimes we forage food out of takeout containers and serve it on paper plates. Three of my kids like to cook with me, the others prefer to do the dishes (well, "prefer" may be a bit generous).

Our family table has been the gossamer that has carried my family and me through illness, divorce, and now, a global pandemic. Cooking and eating together is the only thing that feels remotely "normal" to me, and though they may be loath to admit it, for my kids, too. When the storm is picking up speed, that dinner table is the thing that tethers us, keeping us all from being blown away. It is a quiet thread: you can only see it in a certain light, but it is there, and it is strong.

I imagine living in quarantine is challenging for even the most intact families. Lately I've been wondering how the Bradys would have handled it. I picture card games and family art projects, maybe a musical? If the Bradys had Instagram, Carol would definitely be posting theme dinners of the eight of them dressed in tie-dye or disco outfits. If they had TikTok, there'd be a viral dance routine. They'd post family outings from a beautiful budding forest or a pier somewhere with a sunset in the background.

> When the storm is picking up speed, that dinner table is the thing that tethers us, keeping us all from being blown away.

There are, to be sure, real-life families living much like the Bradys would. I've seen some of their posts: family "chore" charts, picnics, and group workout sessions. I'm happy for them, I really am. But to be clear, A) I do not believe them for a second, and B) If they are for real, those are not my people, and I deeply mistrust them.

That is unfair, I know. But it is honest.

My big aha moment of the past few weeks (aside from the absolute hubris of taking anything at all for granted) is that, as it turns out, I don't think I'd like the Bradys very much if I met them today.

We are most definitely not the Bradys and that's okay. What we are is good enough and even when it's not, there's something inside of all of us that is grateful for the table and optimistic that we'll have the chance to do it all over again tomorrow. There's some comfort in that.

Alison Cayne is the founder of Haven's Kitchen, a cooking school, café, and storefront in New York, and the author of The Haven's Kitchen Cooking School: Recipes and Inspiration to Build a Lifetime of Confidence in the Kitchen.

There Are No Plans to Make, So Why Not Plan Meals?

LAUREN BRAUN COSTELLO

Finding comfort in the mise en place.

Beds in my house are always made and meals are always planned, just as the sun rises and sets and a single sock gets lost each week in the dryer. The scanning of my cupboard and calendar, the conversation I have with myself as mother, chef, organizer in chief, and friend of the farmers' market, is my process. Dinner—and now breakfast and lunch, too, thank you very much COVID-19!—must be plotted out in advance.

What works for me stems both from my personality and profession. I'm a habitual planner who thrives when things are in order. I'm also a natural curator and editor. I like this here and that over there. Order is simultaneously my metronome and my horizon, both a process and an objective, like pilaf or risotto. No wonder I decided to take the leap and become a professional cook nearly two decades ago. What better way to plan, create, curate, edit, repeat, revise, and perfect (or at least attempt to perfect). Cooking is entirely about preparedness—mise en place—the endeavor to execute with the efficiency and proficiency that comes as a result of meticulous planning.

Mise en place literally means "put in place" in French, but it might as well mean "take time to save time." Wash, peel, cut, measure, and select before you begin the cooking process. Set out each measured ingredient—and each tool—ready to play its part. Every recipe begins with the mise en place—two cups of chopped onions, three tablespoons olive oil—so that you know what you need to have ready to begin cooking, to execute the enumerated instructions. Think of meal planning as the mise en place you need to outline not only what you'll be eating but also what you'll need to procure.

Order is simultaneously my metronome and my horizon, both a process and an objective, like pilaf or risotto.

Even as a professional cook, I did not always see the value of routine meal planning. Once I had children, I found the pursuit empowering. Control! Ah, delicious, seductive control. Planning my sons' meals gave me the power to shape and direct not only their days and weeks, but also their lifelong well-being and habits. I could hit a lot of targets and check a lot of boxes with one task. I find that meal planning functions that way: In one fell swoop I can know what I will be eating, what I will be buying (and thus where I need to do the shopping), and ultimately what I will be doing each day, to a degree. I can control only so much, but it's more than a little satisfying to have control at least over all of that.

I remember reading somewhere that in France parents are provided with a monthly menu from the school district that lists both what the children will be served at school each day and a helpful suggestion of what a healthy dinner could be for the corresponding evening. As I remember it, the article read something like this: "If lunch is ratatouille and cabillaud, we recommend perhaps a dinner of buttered noodles and courgettes." *Mais bien sûr* and *mon dieu* all in one. Also, voilà!

That's it! That is the key to planning meals for the family. I looked at it like a math equation: Balance + Variety = Attainable Success.

If school is serving chicken fingers with steamed carrots and rice, then I feel good about a smoothie and muffin for breakfast because lunch features a substantial protein. Dinner, then, can be some fish-and-vegetable dish (roasted, broiled, or sautéed but definitely not fried since that happened at lunch) or pasta and a salad.

Once I approached each day's meal planning with that mindset, the whole week took shape with varied and balanced menus. It wasn't just about the ingredients, but the cooking methods and global flavor profiles, too. My process became an internal dialogue, a conversation I have with myself. "I need a fish here, and a beef there. A ravioli would be perfect Tuesday. The farmers' market is Thursday, so I definitely want to do something with kale and kabocha squash on Friday night. Sunday I can make blintzes because it's leftovers for lunch, and then it's dim sum out for dinner." Planning days into the future helps me to reclaim pockets of time in the present.

As for the future, it is no longer possible to plan more than one week at a time. We are now living in uncharted territory, collectively, in isolation from one another yet miraculously connected through technology. Meal planning is a way to give these chaotic times a sense of structure. It's also a way to commune within our homes and with one another over social media. I've been sharing my meal planning daily on my Instagram feed (@itslaurenofcourse), which has spurred creativity and fostered community, two things that are presently feeding me as much as the food itself. In a world where the safety and health of our loved ones is more fragile than ever and the simple pleasures of quotidian life have been curtailed, planning your next meal might just be the perfect balm.

⊕

Lauren Braun Costello is a cooking instructor, food stylist, and author of multiple books, including The Competent Cook: Essential Tools, Techniques, and Recipes for the Modern At-Home Cook *and* Notes on Cooking.

Food Can Hurt

RENE DENFELD

Before even the age of memory, I knew that food hurt.

We were very poor. My mother drank and forgot to buy food. I'll never forget the taste of the stale saltines I found in the back of otherwise empty cupboards. I must have been very hungry. Each pebble of salt magnified, like the ocean in my mouth.

School lunches were my favorite part of the day: the square of gluey pizza, dotted with fake white cheese. Watery corn. Tuna casserole. Hunger makes you love everything you eat, and then poverty stamps it with shame.

My brother Dennis loved fried bologna. We cut the edges with scissors and fried it quickly, in hot fat. The edges burned and crisped, and we made sandwiches with white bread and the hot grease. Those little Banquet potpies were the greatest treats. By the time I was nine, my mother quit drinking, but we were still poor. By then I had become a connoisseur of the finest generic macaroni and cheese. (It was the now-defunct Western Family brand.)

Later, homeless as a young teen, the rare times I had money—often from panhandling, sometimes from worse—I would gorge. Dozens of dry powdery donuts from the corner store. Packs of cold hot dogs. I often wept as I ate. When life is cracking you open, your hunger bleeds.

A fellow homeless kid turned me on to his favorite poverty meal: a sleeve of Ritz crackers, dipped in a tub of Crisco. We ate uncooked ramen noodles from the packets, crushed with the seasoning packets added, shaking them into our mouths. We were never full.

If you've ever wondered why homeless people can be malnourished and yet overweight, this is why. I was pudgy on the streets, and yet had open sores on my legs from malnutrition. I moved slowly, like I was in a dream.

It was food that rescued me. When I was sixteen I was able to get a work permit, and McDonald's hired me. I washed up in the bathroom before work. I was proud of the rusty-purple uniform. Besides working, the best part was the free daily meal. We got to choose between a Quarter Pounder or chicken nuggets. I always chose the Quarter Pounder. After months of starvation-level nutrients, I could feel that protein hit my veins. The open sores on my legs healed. I gained energy.

Before even the age of memory, I knew that food hurt.

With the income from that job I was able to do what is near impossible anymore: I got a cheap apartment. From there it was a hard but rewarding climb out of poverty to where I am now. My history helps me understand my clients from my justice work, my kids from foster care, and has been the inspiration behind several novels.

I still have mixed and sometimes angry feelings around food. I shop at our local Grocery Outlet because I am a single foster mom on a budget. I hear people sneeringly call it Gross Outlet, as if affordable but perfectly decent food is inherently gross. As if being poor is gross.

Food has been weaponized. We shame mothers for not feeding their kids whatever the popular diet of the moment is, heedless of cost or time. The more women need to work, the more time we demand they spend in the kitchen. I am often contacted by aspiring women authors asking how to fit writing into their parenting schedules. Give up being super mom, I tell them. You don't have to cook dinner every night.

You can almost hear the gasping.

I'm not surprised so many people feel so empty, in such times. We are looking to food for what it cannot do—make us moral, virtuous people. But what makes us moral people is not feeding ourselves. It is feeding others.

If we truly cared about what people ate, we would stop judging and start providing. We would stop the shame game.

When I am feeling sad, or missing my brother, I hunger for fried bologna. I want to cook it in a pan puddled with grease, taking care to cut the edges first. I want to sandwich it between slices of cheap white bread. I want to cry when I eat, knowing the history of people is a history of food, and how we have found ways to make even this act unbearable.

When life is cracking you open, your hunger bleeds.

🕐

Rene Denfeld is the bestselling author of The Child Finder *and* The Butterfly Girl.

It Was Never about the Dough

SONALI DEV

When I perfected my roti, it meant I was finally ready to become a wife.

One of my earliest memories is the smell of fresh rotis roasting in my family's kitchen. Nothing compares to the scent of grain dough as it cooks on an open flame. It's like earth and fire condensed into an aroma that hits your hunger centers just so. If you've smelled baking bread, you know what I mean—now just add to it a hint of embers.

Growing up, I loved watching my mother knead the dough, form it into balls, then roll it into perfect flat circles. She did it every single day. My aunts, my grandmothers—they all did.

As a toddler, when I watched my mother go through her daily ritual, she would hand me a ball of dough to play with. She did this with my children, too. Like me, they'd mold the pliable dough with with the glee of mad scientists. As a young girl, I'd stand by her with my toy-sized rolling pin and mirror her actions. By the time I was a teenager I knew how to knead the dough. I would often make it too sticky and my mother would show me how to add flour to fix it.

I don't remember when my oddly shaped early attempts turned into perfect circles, but at some point my mother began to look on with pride—I even made my father clap the first time I placed a perfect hot one on his plate. What I do remember is that somehow knowing how to do that—to turn flour into bread—equated to my being ready to be a wife.

I'm not from a particularly traditional family, and the patriarchy usually hung around the outskirts of our home; my parents tried to keep it out, even as it pushed in from the world outside. Had I hated being in the kitchen, I don't think my mother would have insisted I learn. Then again maybe I was lured in, seduced by her skill, by the accolades she won at mealtimes. Somewhere along the way the skill got tangled up in being a nurturer and a woman, and then it started to feel like I'd been cheated. The pointed praise of fathers, the casual bragging of mothers. My girlfriends and female cousins were expected to be at least passable at cooking, while the only thing the boys were expected to be passable at was eating, and—wait for it—praising how very fabulous we girls were at it. One of my cousins was once even praised for praising my lovely rotis!

> Somewhere along the way the skill got tangled up in being a nurturer and a woman, and then it started to feel like I'd been cheated.

Truth is, they were lovely. Somehow I was already a good girl by virtue of them. All I could do was try not to dwell on it.

And then I got married. At my first mealtime with my husband's extended family, one of his brothers-in-law declared that my mother-in-law could now relax, since she had a helper. "Isn't it lovely!" said everyone, especially everyone with a Y-chromosome, as they sat there benevolently rejoicing in my mother-in-law's impending freedom from a labor not one of them had ever helped her with.

I did help her, however, deftly spinning dough circles with my married woman's rolling pin. "These are so perfect," my father-in-law remarked, "You could use a circle-drawing compass to trace them." He meant to be generous and encouraging, and he truly was in every aspect of my life, but that sense that somehow I was being slipped something without my knowledge returned. There was something wrong with a picture where men sat at a table and offered not just praise but "constructive" criticism for meals they had no hand in making. It felt like a finely orchestrated farce perfected over centuries and generations.

My mother, a housewife who approached keeping house with the purpose of a CEO running a company, would tell you that this was her job: putting food on the table, spreading joy one taste bud at a time. She'd tell you that the praise was her certificate for excelling at a role she had chosen. I, however, had not chosen that job. I had a more advanced education and career than most of the men who sat there enjoying my rotis and not getting up to help.

> Like so many immigrants before us, we turned to food as our glue. Feeding and being fed became synonymous with love.

Then I moved to the United States, a young immigrant. My husband and I got down to the business of building a life from nothing. Not just graduate degrees and new jobs, but creating community, making family from friendships. Like so many immigrants before us, we turned to food as our glue. Feeding and being fed became synonymous with love.

For the first few years I forgot my discomfort. I rolled dough and watched the perfect circles swell to spheres. Then it started; my ears began to pick out conversations that listed which wives in our circle made rotis and which did not. My ability to look away died a quick death as male friends tendered unsolicited roti-making advice without ever touching a rolling pin. I found myself again with that sense of being taken for a fool.

This sense grew like a slow flood going from connection to connection. All the ways in which I'd been shoved into roles, from being responsible for meals and my home to the care of everyone in my sphere to forcing my feet into heels that made my back hurt to shaving my legs and doing my hair. Things I might enjoy naturally, but I would never know for sure. It all became one.

I stopped making rotis—my very own grand declaration of independence. Fortunately for my husband, who is domestic in many ways but never once considered stepping into the roti-maker's role, the Indian grocery stores in our town started stocking the blameless bread.

Then came the closed stores of this quarantine life, followed by the great bread-making wave. After nearly two decades, I finally broke. Turns out it's like swimming. My body remembered the intricate strokes with the ease of someone indoctrinated young. With that memory returned all the reasons why I had stopped. But I also remembered how much I actually enjoyed it. Was that because there is something magical about turning out perfect bread, or was it because I knew I'd never go back to it as a daily chore? As is the case with anything we've been conditioned to believe about ourselves, I guess I'll never know.

🕐

Sonali Dev is the author of multiple Bollywood-style love stories, including the recent Recipe for Persuasion.

In Provence, Soothed by Goat Yogurt

PHYLLIS GRANT

***In the wee small hours, my mind goes to
a supermarket in the South of France.***

Advice: In the middle of the night, when your unregulated hormones jolt you awake, gently nudge the dog off your legs, flick the sweat off your chest, and consider mentally assembling galettes and salads. This survival technique might help you stave off the ever-present rabbit holes of distress about kids and remote schooling and COVID-19 and racial injustice that, in the deep dark night, feel vast enough to gobble you up. At 3:00 a.m., you will never ever have the answer to anything. So practice what you know.

Flash back to that hot Thursday last July in the South of France. While the rest of your family tours Marseille, cruising in a boat on the bumpy waves, heading toward the cliffs and caves of Les Calanques, you stand alone in the Monoprix grocery store in Saint-Rémy-de-Provence, smiling broadly at the forty-foot span of refrigerator cases filled with French dairy. Nothing fancy or precious. Some local items. Some from up north. Some organic. Some not. Just magnificently abundant. You pile the grocery cart high with six-packs of fromage frais, mini glass jars of goat yogurt, pourable crème fraîche, tubs of fromage blanc, Beurre d'Isigny, and crème fleurette so thick you could cry.

You drive back to the empty house, stand underneath the wisteria, and let the yellow jackets encircle you. The noon heat forces you to sit down and drink crisp, cold rosé. The rules feel different.

Moving quickly, you roll your tart dough out into a jagged circle, giddy as the neon-yellow butter spreads like a spider's web. For the base, you whip together goat yogurt, crème fraîche, crème fleurette, egg, lemon zest, and salt and spread it out evenly over the dough with a butter knife.

Then add some slow-cooked tomatoes from the previous day's lunch. Some chopped herbs. Blobs of ricotta because: why not? A clockwise folding in of the edges.

Egg wash. Extra salt. A quick fix to prevent a leak. And into the oven. The kitchen appliances are unfamiliar so you stick around and peek through the oven window as the tomatoes and whipped dairy bubble and brown and rise and then fall from the bursts of high heat.

At 3:00 a.m., you will never ever have the answer to anything.

While the galette cools, you tuck peach and avocado halves together on a large dinner plate, filling all of their bellies with garlic oil, pickled onions, and Champagne vinegar. Then a bit of parsley and coarse salt. A thwack of lemon zest. And then splat. Splat. Splat. Crème fraîche everywhere.

If you aren't asleep by now, just get up and start cooking.

Crème Fraîche

I splash this over pasta, stews, avocado toasts, and tacos. I mix it into green goddess dressing, tart bases, and pesto. It is a wonderful replacement for sour cream. It's a lovely way to cut the sweet intensity of a cake or pie. Once you have it in your life, you will be tempted to use it every single day.

    1 cup heavy cream
    2 tablespoons buttermilk

Pour the heavy cream and the buttermilk into a jar with an available lid. Stir just to mix. Put on the lid. Leave it on the counter. The thickening and souring take anywhere from 1 to 4 days. The hotter your kitchen, the faster it will go. Stir and taste every 12 hours or so. Once it's to your liking, store it covered in the fridge for up to a month. I make this every two weeks. Every six months or so, a batch doesn't work. If it smells or tastes like blue cheese, toss it and start over.

You roll your tart dough into a jagged circle, giddy as the neon-yellow butter spreads like a spider's web.

🕐

Recipe from *Everything is Under Control: A Memoir With Recipes* by Phyllis Grant[1]
Phyllis Grant is a three-time Saveur Food Blog Award finalist for her blog, Dash and Bella. *Her latest book is* Everything Is Under Control: A Memoir with Recipes.

What I Saw at Your Kid's Birthday Party

LAURA HANKIN

Confessions of a children's musician
for the one percent.

I used to sing at children's birthday parties. As an aspiring writer and performer, I needed a flexible day job. And after a series of false starts as a flash mob coordinator (yes, that was a real thing) and an assistant to a psychoanalyst who needed therapy of his own, I discovered the lucrative world of kids' entertainment.

On any given weekend, I lugged my guitar and a bag of egg shakers across New York City like a wandering minstrel, entertaining wealthy babies in their gorgeous apartments. After I finished singing, the mothers would often invite me to stick around for a plate of party food. It might have been more dignified to graciously decline and get the hell out, but here's the thing about me: I am incapable of turning down free food.

So I'd load up a plate of hors d'oeuvres—deviled eggs, toothpicks of caprese. Sometimes, the parents had gone for full-on catered meals, and I'd ladle spoonfuls of chana masala onto my plate, or cut a piece of rich, steaming lasagna. And always, there was cake: flourless chocolate tortes from fancy bakeries or ultra-sweet concoctions with the _Paw Patrol_ pups drawn on top in unnaturally bright icing.

The free food created a problem, though. While I ate it, I had to stay and hang out. The parents had hired me to entertain, and I had served my purpose. Now who was I supposed to talk to? Should I continue to play with the children even though I was off the clock? Or did I dare talk to the adults? I felt as awkward as a middle schooler, scanning the cafeteria for a table where I belonged. Generally, I just gobbled my food as quickly as I could, and watched the party play out.

In the noisy, sticky crowd, the mothers whirled, holding a champagne glass in one hand and wiping the crumbs off their child's face with the other. The celebrations they threw for their children were often lavish, packed with eighty of their closest friends like miniature weddings. Sometimes, in the midst of playing perfect hostess, their frustration came through, frustration with partners who weren't helping enough, or with children who wouldn't let them finish their conversations.

I wondered, as I devoured my Brie and crackers, if my life would ever look like theirs. If someday I would have a husband and we'd put on our finest clothes to celebrate our one-year-old. I wasn't sure if I'd be able to afford to have children on an artist's salary. And maybe I didn't want them anyway—how would they affect all the big dreams I had for my career? Sure, at the moment I was spending more time traipsing around to these birthday parties than being creative, often too exhausted by the time I got back home to do much more than collapse in front of the TV, but still. I felt that if I were to have children, I would need to establish myself first so that people would miss me when I took time away and be willing to accommodate me when I came back. And yet the years were floating by and I seemed to be getting no closer to establishing anything at all.

On any given weekend, I lugged my guitar and a bag of egg shakers across New York City like a wandering minstrel, entertaining wealthy babies in their gorgeous apartments.

I was in my mid-twenties when I started doing these parties, but as my thirtieth birthday drew closer, the mothers started to look different to me. Sometimes they still grimaced in frustration. And sometimes they laughed with pure delight, so lucky and happy to be exactly where they were.

As I shoveled down some chicken fingers at an "On the Farm"-themed birthday party that would turn out to be one of my last, I finally realized I couldn't do this forever. I wanted a life where I was building something. I didn't need to throw the event of the season for my one-year-old. But maybe I did want, someday, to be the mother offering a plate. Maybe I wanted to shovel down food not because I didn't know what to do with myself, but because I had so much to do and needed to get back to it.

> I was in my mid-twenties when I started doing these parties, but as my thirtieth birthday drew closer, the mothers started to look different to me.

I finished the cold chicken tender and wiped my fingers on a balloon-patterned napkin. I waved goodbye to the busy, whirling woman who had hired me. "Thank you!" she called out. Then she returned to her life and I walked out the door.

🕐

Laura Hankin is a performer and author of the debut novel Happy and You Know It.

To Papayas, With Love
COURTNEY MAUM

**Quelling my pandemic fears in Mexico,
one fruit at a time.**

I stood at the bottom of the cobbled driveway contemplating the desiccated orange halves and yellowed husks of corn below the thorn trees and I knew that my life was about to change, in a big way.

No more Western Mexico. No more scorpions hiding behind my daughter's pillow. No more hauling compost a quarter mile through the jungle so the coatis didn't rip through the kitchen window screens to get at our garbage. With the exception of the scorpions, these realizations brought me sadness, not relief.

I was in my sixth week in Careyes, a small coastal community in the rural state of Jalisco on Mexico's Pacific Coast. I'd come to Mexico on March 8 with my husband and young daughter to promote the Spanish edition of my latest novel, *Costalegre*, and then COVID-19 hit—or rather, COVID-19 escalated—to a degree that presented an urgent question: should we stay or should we go?

There were tons of considerations on the "stay" side and only two on the "go" end: "Wi-Fi" and "our cat." But our cat was safe in Connecticut with friends who were happy to have him. As for the Wi-Fi, the Internet was zipping panic through a billion routers, so that left zero reasons to leave the place we were.

A free home in paradise, infinity pool privileges, all of these were no-brainer reasons to stay put, but one of the more serious ones was access to fresh food. In the pictures my phone brought me (dispatches I accessed by hanging over a banister situated on a cliff to get one bar of network) I saw supermarkets emptied of toilet paper, body soap, poultry and meat products, all produce gone but durian, nowhere to buy flour. I live in a rural part of the Northeast where the closest grocery store is a struggling Stop & Shop. Stadium-sized, glacially air-conditioned, and staffed almost entirely with self-checkout terminals, it is a shopping experience so depressing that I listen to a sex podcast when I go there to distract myself from the fact that even the ripest vegetables look like they came to our grocery store to die.

In Mexico, I developed an orange juice addiction that felt like the start of an affair.

As a self-employed writer married to an independent film director, we survive the ups and downs of a creative life by spending carefully, but in our corner of northwestern Connecticut, even a rote trip to the grocery store ends in a three digit receipt. From a culinary perspective, returning during COVID-19 would mean spending money we weren't earning on food we didn't enjoy. Though I don't consider myself a foodie, I do think of food and beverage as a great reward system: you nail your presentation, there's a plate of carbonara pasta waiting on the other side. This habit of equating food with gratification is problematic, childish. It's one of the reasons I didn't feel up to the task of homeschooling my daughter for the payoff of frozen cauliflower florets.

So we stayed in Mexico. We stayed among the papayas that ripened on slim trunks, the limes greening on branches, the mangos weighing down the broad leaves of the trees that dutifully bore them. Although we didn't have an oven, a short car ride took us to a corner store where a husband and wife team pressed out fresh tortilla rounds, the heat of the wax-paper package a replacement for another human's hand. In Mexico, I developed an orange juice addiction that felt like the start of an affair. Unsustainable and tenuous though this new love was, I nonetheless kept at it: four oranges squeezed into an elixir of optimism and hope each morning, a dose of vitamins that built a wall against my dread.

We were tasked with jobs in our tropical shelter: my daughter spotted scorpions and my husband caught them (it pains me to say "killed" although that was the end goal), and I cooked and walked the compost into the jungle every day. This chore was performed in the grueling heat of day's end or the mosquito rave of nightfall, and while my epidermis didn't win in either scenario, I came to love the daily descents that gave me the opportunity to appreciate the food that nourished my family and eased my anxious mind. My latest book tour was canceled, all my speaking engagements, nixed. Deals that would have brought me income had vanished into thin air. When these realizations edged at me, an avocado doused in sea salt and olive oil was a balm to my new fears. When another day came to a close without a family breakdown, we barbecued pineapple with a pinch of lime. When the sun came up and it was time for us to be on top of one other once again, cuts of ripe papaya gave us fortitude—and fiber—for the day ahead.

And so it was that my compost duties became a cherished ritual; the dumping of egg shells, candles to an altar. The scattered orange halves, the wrinkled limes, the slicks of papaya wet as dolphin's skin, with every remnant that tumbled out of the plastic compost bowl that I carried, I gave thanks for the pause button that Mexico had given us; the incredible opportunity to take time, reflect, reset.

Eventually, however, the abundance of fresh produce could not make up for the lack of Internet in our jungle house. With nowhere to purchase books and mail delivery impossible, we'd run out of materials and activities to homeschool our daughter with, and I couldn't teach any of the online classes that were keeping my fellow writers sane. Our decision to leave was made easier by the fact that our hostess had found someone who wanted to rent her entire place as a "pandemic escape" for two thousand dollars a night.

We purchased a homeward ticket for the fourth of May and we got on a plane, and then we got on another plane, and both planes arrived where they were supposed to, at the time that they were supposed to, with 15 percent of their seats filled. There wasn't any food or beverage service in-flight, but we were handed a gift bag containing a single bottle of water by hands wrapped in plastic gloves. In the checked baggage below us, we carried clothes worn by two months of dust and sunshine alongside a six-pack of toilet paper that we'd bought before the flight.

It was time to face our new reality. The home we would return to had been irrevocably changed. I had no idea what lay in store for me or for my family when we got off the plane. I didn't know what items would be left in the picked-over aisles at Stop & Shop. But I knew that we had been tremendously fortunate to enjoy the gift of isolation in a place where fruit fell from the trees only to split open and create new trees again.

🕑

Courtney Maum is the author of multiple books, including the novels Touch *and* Costalegre, *and the nonfiction guide* Before and After the Book Deal.

The Weight of It All
ZIBBY OWENS

In quarantine, all my old body insecurities came roaring back.

The only reason I bought a scale recently was for my younger children's telemedicine checkups with their pediatrician. Before I could prop the kids up on my desk and have them "open wide" into my desktop's camera, I would need to record their height and weight to have on hand for the appointments. It seemed simple enough. I ordered the same type of old-fashioned, floor-model scale that looked exactly like the one I had in high school and that had followed me for twenty years afterward.

The scale and I have had a fraught relationship since I was nine years old. That was when, according to my mother, I told her I was upset about how much larger my thighs were than all the other girls' at school with their string-bean legs. Sitting at the breakfast table in her bathrobe, smoking a Vantage Ultra and eating half a grapefruit before heading off to Gilda's exercise class, this five-foot-two, petite, toned woman sprang into action. She knew just how to fix this problem.

She bestowed upon me her treasured, dog-eared copy of the book *Calories and Carbohydrates* and taught me how to scan the tiny number lines for each food. I diligently measured half a cup of orange juice over the kitchen sink in my uniform jumper each morning before writing down the calories and then heading off to fourth grade. I remember rushing into my little brother's room one night when my mom was tucking him in and proudly announcing that I had two pieces of great news: I had swallowed my first pill (something for my allergies) and I had successfully stayed under 1,200 calories for the day.

The real test, of course, was seeing if the scale had gone down. Once a week, I would stand in my mother's bathroom, which smelled like Pond's cold cream and Nivea lotion, and step on her doctor's scale. I'd nudge the black markers right or left until the pendulum balanced and stopped wavering up and down. I always wanted to push it farther and father left. Never mind that I was still growing. I wanted to fit in with my waiflike friends. I wanted my body to look like theirs; perhaps then I would be completely accepted.

I couldn't control the chaos of having twins. I couldn't absorb the shock of going from being an overachiever to spending my days on the playroom floor, longing for the time when I could just get to sleep again. But losing weight gave me a quantifiable goal.

For the next thirty years, I tried every diet and exercise fad imaginable while ricocheting up and down five, ten, fifteen, or twenty pounds, all within a tight range like a Ping-Pong ball going back and forth over the net of a faded table. Atkins. Step aerobics. Carbohydrate Addicts. Tae bo. A clinic on 63rd Street that gave me "vitamins." HIIT. It was never enough. If only I could lose a few pounds, I could remove the shackle of shame I felt was constantly wrapped around my neck like a Parisian woman's scarf. I was embarrassed by the outward display of my inner mess. I wanted to at least look like I had it all together when inside I was worried, anxious, and trying to find my place in the world.

After business school in 2003, I became a Weight Watchers addict and adhered so strictly to the program that I lost thirty pounds and even became a Leader, running meetings all over New York City to spread the gospel. I counted Points and wrote down every food I ate for almost ten years, through three pregnancies and four kids. I couldn't get over the joy I felt that there actually was a solution! Something that worked. I couldn't control the chaos of having twins. I couldn't absorb the shock of going from being an overachiever to spending my days on the playroom floor, longing for the time when I could just get to sleep again. But losing weight gave me a quantifiable goal. Something for me. Something to aspire to when grades and salary and all other external measures of success suddenly evaporated.

I was trying to find that elusive sense of control, that hook to tether myself to, and then punishing myself when I couldn't pull it off.

Yet losing all that weight wasn't good for me physically; my hair started falling out, I stopped getting my period, and I was always cold. One doctor I consulted even said, "Your body just isn't made to be this skinny, and that's okay." In retrospect, trying to control my intake and keep my body looking its best was the way I tried to cope as my first marriage fell apart, and I felt powerless to save it. The inner turmoil was on full display. I ate my feelings. I structured my diet because I could control that more than I could control my life. I ate in secret to cope with the things that went on in my home that I didn't discuss.

At some point during the last five years, after my divorce and in my new relationship with Kyle, who became my husband, I made a delicate peace with my body and started focusing on work instead. I stopped weighing myself unless my zippers strained as I yanked them up and I knew I had to regroup. I accepted that to eat the way I wanted without expending an inordinate amount of energy "watching it," I would be three or four sizes larger than my goal weight.

And then the pandemic hit. I felt enormously lucky to be healthy and financially secure when so many others were suffering from the start. My first thoughts were more about food scarcity and the nation's food supply system than my jeans. I was so scared and nervous as we hunkered down that I couldn't eat that much. I was in survival mode. I threw my energy into helping buoy the literary community when I wasn't taking care of my four kids and cleaning the house. For exercise, my teen daughter asked me to do a YouTube "summer shred" workout program with her. I'll do anything for her, even crunches and burpees, so we did it daily.

And then the scale arrived.

I took it out of the box and placed it on my cold bathroom floor. My little guy hopped right on.

"Mom, get on with me!" he said excitedly. "Come on!"

I hadn't been on a scale in months, but I had a number in mind (the high end of my Ping-Pong range) that I fully expected to see.

I got on the scale with my son and quickly did the math. Wait, that couldn't be right.

"Honey, let me try this alone for a second, okay?"

I gasped.

I stared down at a number that was ten pounds higher than I expected. A number I'd only seen while pregnant. And here I thought I'd lost weight!

All the old demons came racing out, taunting me. You're fat! You're lazy! You're pathetic! You're out of control! How could you! The number was far above my "before" weight when I started Weight Watchers almost twenty years ago.

I backed away from the scale and ushered my son out of the suddenly toxic bathroom.

That night, I began aggressively stuffing my face with food, perversely punishing myself with the same weapon that had gotten me into this mess. I started obsessing about my weight, the foods I was eating, what I "should" and "shouldn't" consume, scarfing down cookie after cookie at night when everyone else in the house was finally sleeping.

Naturally, several days later, my clothes felt tight for the first time in months.

I was falling back into my self-punishing habits, like an armchair sliding back into the well-worn depressions in the carpet after being temporarily pushed aside. I almost couldn't believe it: after all these years, the same feelings were still there, ever-present.

I can see now that I was reaching for my telltale crutch, the one I routinely steadied myself with in times of stress and uncertainty. And what is a pandemic if not a time of extreme stress and uncertainty? I was trying to find that elusive sense of control, that hook to tether myself to, and then punishing myself when I couldn't pull it off.

It was a sobering reminder that achieving balance is a lifelong journey with plenty of backslides along the way.

Soon after, the craziness, busyness, and fear of day-to-day COVID-19 life overtook me again. (What about camp?! A new disease affecting children?!? Should we move?) But this time, I handled things a bit differently.

My food rumination waned: I started to plan. I got caught up in life again, in helping my kids and my community, in looking outward.

Zibby Owens is a writer and mother of four in New York City. She is a literary advocate and the creator and host of the award-winning literary podcast Moms Don't Have Time to Read Books. *She runs a literary salon with author events, a virtual book club, and a daily* Z-IGTV *live author interview series.*

Baking Challah to Connect
BETH RICANATI, MD

think it is fair to say that getting my hands sticky and covered with flour in a bowl of dough saved my life. Three kids, a career as a physician, a husband who worked full time: it all left me overwhelmed, burned out—before that was even a term bantered about in my profession. I was having difficulty staying safely on the hamster wheel that I unwittingly created for myself.

Fortunately, stopping one day, staring in disbelief at six ingredients arrayed on my kitchen counter, I began—unbeknownst to me at the time—a journey toward a healthier life. As they say, doctor, heal thyself, and well over 1,200 loaves of challah bread later, I can say I found a way to do just that.

I thought it was a great idea to have three kids in four years. Truly. Twenty years of education and this was my grand insight. Alas, not so grand in hindsight: the costs to my well-being were steep. Most nights, I collapsed into bed after making sure everyone was fed and bathed and read to and the dishes were done and permission slips signed and snacks packed and medical journals rearranged in the same growing pile in the corner. Never mind the exercise that I was supposed to be getting or the extra reading that I should have been doing. When we moved to Cleveland (where our third child was born) from New York City, into a house with actual closet space, I discovered Target as my ubiquitous source for diapers and pull-ups. Better yet, how fabulous was it that Target had a deal with designer Isaac Mizrahi, and I could get a cool sundress along with all those baby supplies. I had arrived, and while the diapers eventually went away, the dress survived for years.

I remained on this hamster wheel until I couldn't keep it up anymore, and finding time to brush my teeth twice a day actually seemed like a luxury. Then challah entered my life: I found that stopping and diving into this ancient ritual was the secret way to finding a way to be present again.

I started making challah over a decade ago at the suggestion of a friend, and I make this special bread—bread that nourishes us both physically and spiritually—every Friday. Initially, it was to be a one-time thing, just for the holidays that year. But the experience was so transformative that I continued to make it weekly. I make it by myself or sometimes with my friends. I make it in my home, and I make it when I'm traveling (I used to bring packets of yeast with me; I've since discovered how easy it is to get the ingredients locally). It has become my Friday ritual. Research demonstrates that the tactile arts help to reduce anxiety and help us to be present; done as a community, tactile arts—making challah in my case—are a terrific way to combat loneliness (a rising epidemic in America). As a new mother and a young physician, I had not appreciated how alone I could feel surrounded by so many people. In hindsight, making challah was just the prescription I needed. And now, as we all come together to combat the growing coronavirus pandemic, paying heed to our mental health becomes even more important. There are many ways to feel good in times like these; making bread is but one. I find the meditative aspect of kneading dough therapeutic.

One loaf at time, we are building community together across this country of ours.

So moved by what I had learned, I wrote about it. *Braided: A Journey of a Thousand Challahs* was published in the fall of 2018 (She Writes Press). Turns out, I am not alone in my feelings for the need for connection and ritual. Since publication, readers have been sending me their gorgeous challah pictures after reading *Braided*, often accompanied by their own story. Stories of friendship and loss, stories of breast cancer survival, and simply joy in finding challah. One loaf at a time, we are building community together across this country of ours. We are connecting, forging bonds. Our identifying labels don't seem to matter: rural versus urban-dwelling; Jewish or non-Jewish; male or female. Making bread, leaning into an ancient ritual, being present. This is what matters. So go ahead, get out some flour, eggs, oil, salt, sugar, and yeast. Set aside some time, and make some challah. The recipe is at the beginning of the book. When you take those gorgeous loaves out of the oven, snap a photo and send it my way.

I remained on this hamster wheel until I couldn't keep it up anymore, and finding time to brush my teeth twice a day actually seemed like a luxury. Then challah entered my life.

I'd love to add it to the growing photo gallery on my website, www.BethRicanatiMD.com.

P.S. If you actually have any leftovers, it makes great French toast the next day!

⊕

Beth Ricanati, MD, is the debut author of Braided: A Journey of a Thousand Challahs. *A physician, Beth bakes challah weekly.*

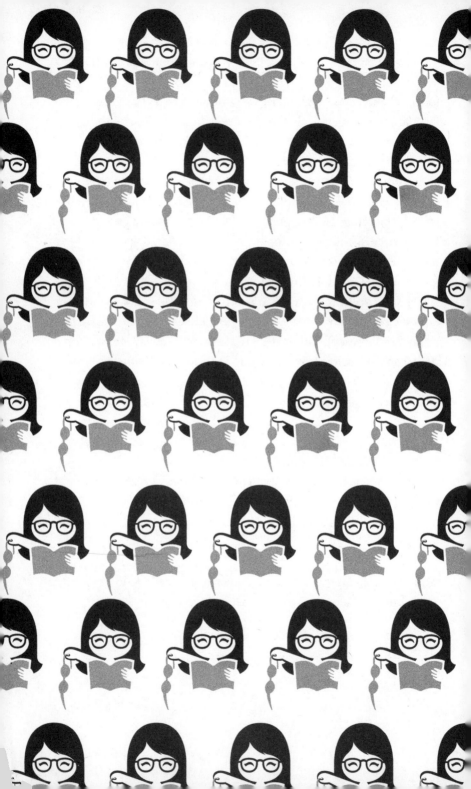

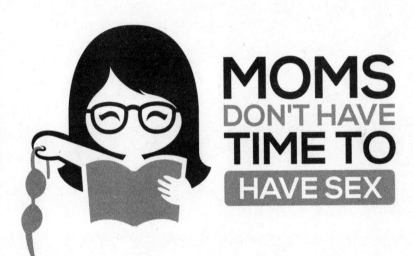

Forget Date Night—Try Date Day

LISA BARR

Why sunlight is the best aphrodisiac.

A little glimpse into my former, pre-coronavirus life: Every day, after the kids left for school, my husband and I would meet at a nearby café for twenty minutes. No phone calls would be answered, no meetings scheduled, no emails replied to. During "coffee time," our sole focus was always our relationship. These morning dates were more than just an easy way to satisfy my craving for a grande extra hot mocha with whip (although, that was usually there, too). In those precious, stolen moments, in a crowded café filled with busy people going about their own pre-pandemic lives, I felt seen. My husband and I treasured those daily opportunities to remember why we chose each other in the first place.

Our day dates felt a little hot, a little secretive, and yes, sometimes a little naughty. Like we were sneaking around. Once, a woman approached us and said, "I see you two here every morning, holding hands. I know it's none of my business, but are you having an affair?"

"Yes," I laughed. "An affair with my husband."

We are not newlyweds. We have been together seventeen years, each our second marriage, with three daughters between us. (Our home could also be referred to as "Drama Central.") We've had our fair share of problems. And yet, our relationship is still full of passion and love. Having learned from our pasts, we know exactly what it takes to keep a relationship intact—and also what can break it.

I'm here to tell you: "date night" is bullshit. Yes, it's a celebrated tradition among many couples, but as I see it, it's just another Hallmark holiday, manufactured and forced, like Valentine's Day. For many couples, "date night" comes with a long list of requirements: Make a dinner reservation, find an expensive babysitter who will (hopefully) put the kids to bed, dress up, force adult conversation, and then cap off the night with sex. It's no wonder that "date night" rarely seems to live up to all of the glimmering, high expectations that surround it. If you ignore your marriage six days a week, one night out cannot erase the distance that has been created.

Plus, by the end of a long day, many women (especially those with young kids), would rather have hot sleep than hot sex.

Our marriage works better when we date during the day. "Date day" presses pause on all of life's minutia. For a few moments, we're able to see one another out in the sunlight, before being drained by the inevitable demands the day will bring. For us, "date day" doesn't just stop when we finish our coffee. Throughout the day, even when it seems like there isn't enough time, I let my husband know that I am thinking about him. And he has learned to do the same. This is where emojis come in handy! With a tap of a thumb, I can send a heart or a kiss or an eggplant to tell him he is on my mind. This is *sexy*. This is *connection*. This is *foreplay*.

Of course, there are certainly days when we have our coffee time and emoji exchanges, and at the end of the day I would still rather check out and watch a TV show by myself. Yet our established routine takes resentment out of the picture.

Admittedly, the recent "shelter-in-place" orders have created a bit of an obstacle for our "date day" routine. This virus is a serious cockblocker. There have been countless moments during this endless lockdown in which I have wanted to slay my husband. And there are none of our usual emoji exchanges, because he's literally sitting right next to me. (Did you know that during quarantine, a top divorce attorney said there has been a 50 percent rise in filings? I hate to say it, but I'm not surprised.)

> Believe me, my husband has never looked as hot to me as he does unloading the dishwasher.

As the days began to blur together—is it Wednesday or Saturday?—I realized that my marriage needed a boost of vitamin A. A, as in attention. As in ASAP. Without our consistent day dates, that absence of resentment that I was so proud of before started to build. Competition (I did this, you didn't do that) replaced romance, and we became blind to one another, even in the same damn room. We knew we needed to regroup to recover our mojo.

Now, we wake up before the kids. We shower, put on clean clothes, go for a drive, order curbside coffee from our favorite café, and take a long beach walk (properly distanced, of course). We divide and conquer the dishes, the laundry, the meals, the house details. Believe me, my husband has never looked as hot to me as he does unloading the dishwasher.

We made 5:00 p.m. our official, no-matter-what happy hour. Bourbon for two—yes, please. We've established boundaries in our home, boundaries with our kids, and boundaries with each other. The stupid fights that start over nothing have ceased because we've given ourselves the chance to thwart the bullets before they fly.

"Honey," I said earlier today. "I'm losing it. Totally losing it. I can't write. I can't get a grip."

Because we've practiced, he listened.

When I finally finished my rant, he said, "I hear you and I know exactly what you need. Go. Get out of here. My office is totally empty. Take some time to get your stuff done. Stay off your phone. I've got the laundry. I'll cover the kids, the dog, all the shit you do."

Full stop right here. This guy is so getting laid.

Therein lies the power of "date day." Whether it's back in real life, or throughout this apocalyptic, altered existence: it's not about saving up all your romance ammo for a designated special occasion. Being seen in real-time on a daily basis is a powerful aphrodisiac—a daily supplement necessary for any relationship to survive, and ultimately thrive.

> If you ignore your marriage six days a week, one night out cannot erase the distance that has been created.

⊕

Lisa Barr is the award-winning author of novels The Unbreakables *and* Fugitive Colors.

Here's How Long It Takes to Have Good Sex

RACHEL BERTSCHE

Busy parents, rejoice!

Here's the thing about sex: it doesn't need to take that long.

During my first year of parenthood—certainly for the first few months—sex was off the table for practical reasons: it hurt, the doctor said I couldn't, and I was nursing what seemed like every twenty minutes. Eventually the doctor gave me the all clear. ("Do you want me to say you need more time?" he asked me at my six-week checkup. "Lot of mothers do . . . but you're probably better off to rip off the Band-Aid.") And yet, sex was still a rare event. We were both exhausted. I felt unsexy, still adjusting to this new body that had carried and delivered a small human, and then another one.

As our kids grew up, not much changed. Any attempt at a spontaneous make out was met by kids screaming, "Gross! Get away!" Nights of intimacy were scheduled days in advance, after comparing calendars to find the most convenient evening. Whenever we did do it, we'd find ourselves, afterward, wondering why we'd put it off so long. Still, knowing better didn't mean doing better, and fitting sex into our hectic lives continued to feel daunting. We spent our evenings playing Candy Land, rushing toward bath time, collapsing from exhaustion. Time escaped us.

As I began research for my book, *The Kids Are in Bed: Finding Time for Yourself in the Chaos of Parenting*, I came across some numbers that I found comforting. A survey asked sex therapists how long good sex should last. Turns out, according to the experts, the desirable duration of sex is only seven to thirteen minutes. Three to seven is adequate! Any more than thirteen minutes? Too long.

I was raised on a diet of rom-coms and *Beverly Hills 90210*, which means I always believed romantic evenings were long and passionate and involved refueling over Chinese takeout (eaten in bed and from the carton) before getting tangled up in the sheets again. Obviously, I learned long before having kids that sex doesn't actually look like it does in the movies, but I held on to an idea that "quickies"—while convenient and sometimes rebelliously exciting—weren't good sex.

> I always believed romantic evenings were long and passionate and involved refueling over Chinese takeout . . .

And then here comes science to the rescue! Sure, foreplay and cuddling are real and wonderful activities, when you've got the time. But if you don't, and you still want to keep that flame lit, it's nice to know that a ten-minute romp isn't shortchanging anyone. Because the real problem with sex after kids isn't that we don't do it for long enough, it's that we don't do it at all. We get so mired in the relentless pace of parenting that we don't connect with our partners outside of "it's your turn to change the diaper" or "did you remember to sign the camp permission slip?"

It's too easy, in parenthood, to forget that there was a time, before any offspring invaded the picture, when you wanted to rip each other's clothes off. During my book research, I came across Dr. Mary Andres, a clinical psychologist and couples counselor who specializes in sexuality. She explained that a common complaint among people with "amicable divorces" is a loss of passion. She said, "I've had people say 'He's the best dad ever and I can't imagine divorcing him, but I'm not attracted to him anymore,' and those are sad stories."

I don't want my marriage to be another sad anecdote for a sex researcher to tell a journalist, or a cautionary tale a couples therapist uses to scare her patients. But the "keep the spark alive" advice I find in magazines—text him a sexy photo during the day! Give each other a massage to get in the mood!—seems to be for people with far less on their to-do lists, or maybe who have no kids at all. My four-year-old and my six-year-old use my phone a lot, and they know how to access the photos. I don't need them stumbling on an awkward "sexy pic" I sent in an attempt to pique their father's interest.

> The real problem with sex after kids isn't that we don't do it for long enough, it's that we don't do it at all . . .

What I do need is something practical. What I do need is to understand what qualifies as "enough" during this season of our lives when the margins continue to shrink. One day, we'll have time to relish in all of the tiny moments that lead up to a big explosion. But for now, sex can be short and sweet—less time than a round of Candy Land, and way more fun.

🕐

Rachel Bertsche is a journalist and bestselling author of multiple books, including the recent The Kids Are in Bed: Finding Time for Yourself in the Chaos of Parenting.

When I Got Coronavirus, My Husband Became My Wife

KARMA BROWN

From my sickbed, I coached him on how to keep the household running.

When I got married fifteen years ago, we were still in the place where Dr. Phil's cutesy advice for marital success and happiness—divide your household tasks into "pink" and "blue" jobs—was delivered unironically and without immediate social backlash.

At the time I first heard this guidance, I was a newlywed, we were childless, and it seemed both practical and manageable. Not to mention, "pink" and "blue" distinctions fell mostly in line with our personal preferences (I liked to cook, my husband did not; he could hang pictures, I sucked at making things level; neither of us was overjoyed by garbage duties, but we agreed he would do that if I did groceries . . .). For some time, this arrangement worked just as Dr. Phil said it would—stuff got done, and everyone was happy (enough) about it.

And then we had a child, and my "pink" tasks exploded. Our house felt perpetually untidy, no matter how much I buzzed around in between tummy time and round-the-clock breastfeeding. Our daughter's birth also coincided with my husband starting his business. In Canada we are fortunate to have twelve-months of maternity leave (or nine months of paternity leave), which is a wonderful perk, but also meant I had (hypothetically) more time to double down on pink tasks. Suddenly, all the cooking, cleaning, and childcare fell to me. It was hard not to resent my husband during those first few months as I fantasized about going back to work. Taking a shower solo and drinking still-hot coffee felt like distant memories.

Before having a child, I had only watched mothers from afar with passing curiosity. Until I became one, I didn't appreciate how significantly my life would change—and how little my husband's would. In 2015, 70 percent of mothers participated in the workforce, and about 40 percent were their family's primary breadwinner. At the same time, women today are putting in more childcare hours than they did in 1965, despite also working nearly three times the number of hours they did then.

When I agreed to this pink/blue divide all those years ago I was a small "f" feminist. Today, and especially as a mother, I'm a capital "R" Raging one.

I hadn't understood these nuances of motherhood, or how (in general) society continues to expect women—even those who work as many hours as their partners—to handle the "pink" things, like childcare (and right now during this pandemic, homeschooling). Ali Wong, a comedian who finds plenty of great material for her shows in society's view of mothers and women, talked about how when she came back to work people couldn't stop asking, but . . . who's taking care of the baby? To which she retorted, the TV!

I have a busy career, yet as the one who works from home, I also continue to handle most household tasks because on paper it makes sense. Groceries; cooking and meal planning; most of the logistics when it comes to our child—including being the one to drop work when she's sick, fall to me. I also manage the "emotional labor," like birthday presents, gift cards for teachers, and neighborhood meal trains.

Though I actively agreed to all of this, albeit somewhat naively, I was forced to confront the decision about a year ago. I had declared a (one-time) strike on dinner, and my daughter said, "But that's your job!" A flurry of emotions hit me: panic, frustration, anger, resolve. That night my husband made scrambled eggs, and I explained to my daughter I was not uniquely skilled at cooking (or any other "pink" tasks) because I was a woman. How, yes, our house was divided up a touch stereotypically when it came to gender roles, but that was due to logistics versus our belief system. I realized that night I hadn't lost my voice, I had simply forgotten how to use it.

During the early days of this global pandemic, when life as we knew it came to a screeching halt, I found myself quite sick with a probable case of COVID-19. When I was unable to get off the couch for nearly two weeks, my former blue-job-focused husband had to pivot. He had been forced to temporarily close his businesses to help mitigate the spread, so luckily he was home at the time. For most of those few weeks he took on everything, including all the cooking. I coached him through recipes from my sickbed and he kept our household running, now tuned in to the realities of being a work-at-home parent (children are mess tornadoes). When I recovered, I noted an interesting shift in our marriage: our formerly divided tasks were now in one bucket. Some eleven weeks into lockdown we are a purple-hued household, and it's hard not to see this as a positive by-product of quarantine life.

This won't be true for everyone, as it's estimated women will lose their jobs at a three-to-one ratio compared to men due to this pandemic. My own story likely has a few more chapters, because with no school for the foreseeable future and a husband who will be going back to work, I will soon be trying to work and parent simultaneously once again.

When I agreed to this pink/blue divide all those years ago I was a small "f" feminist. Today, and especially as a mother, I'm a capital "R" Raging one. Raising a young daughter in these times means my husband and I can't be flippant as her role models. Our girl is watching, listening, and learning. I do hope she'll be part of a generation that eschews these stereotypes once and for all, but in the meantime, we'll be seeing more Dad-made dinners on the menu at our house.

🕐

Karma Brown is a journalist and bestselling author of multiple books. Her most recent is the novel Recipe for A Perfect Wife.

Your Orgasm Could Save Your Marriage

V. C. CHICKERING

I've always felt that sex should be fun, like dancing or badminton. Something to look forward to. It's free, requires minimal gear, and better yet, demands no season pass. Wouldn't your life be easier if you enjoyed it?

Men have reached glorious climax, practically each and every time, since the dawn of mankind. Fast-forward to the 1970s, when women collectively demanded, "Enough of this. We want ours, too." Enter a kajillion books, *Cosmopolitan* articles, pamphlets, "personal massagers," Esther Perel, and TED talks about women's desire. And here we are in 2020. Has your partner sought it out? Have they glanced at a diagram lately? Some have. But most? Yeah, no.

Once upon a time you wanted to rip his clothes off, marinating in your hormones and desire. Then, around eighteen to twenty-four months in, those sweaty impulses withered. But he was a good guy with a solid job and your parents liked him, so you tied the knot and bought the two-and-a-half bath. Here you are, now, three kids in. And there he is, over on the couch, because a myriad of social forces are endlessly inserting themselves, wedging too much space between you and your sex lives. Enter the infamous "rough patch," code for: we rarely sleep together anymore. Why? Because there's not enough time? I don't buy it. Maybe it's just not fun for you.

You deserve more than a tepid comfort zone. You're making it work, because you're a woman and that's what we do. We make things work. Perhaps you've convinced yourself that sex was never really your "thing," and now it really isn't. But it still could be. In the same way you research tutors, coaches, and summer camps, it's high time you researched your own orgasm.

Type "tips for better female orgasm" into your Google search bar. I dare you. Then read up! Because it is your job to know how to please your body just as much as it is your partner's. Ask your closest girlfriends what works for them. See this as an investment in your emotional and physical health—an investment that will simultaneously fortify your family. Believe me, claiming your orgasm could very well save your marriage.

You're making it work, because you're a woman and that's what we do.

Fun in bed yields a close, viable connection. You two are the architects of your marriage and convincing yourself he doesn't need sex when he very much wants it is a doomed path. Your relational chasm will only widen. The tension will only increase. After all, you're ignoring a very horny elephant in the room.

How can you turn the ship around?

Try saying, "Hey, honey. I want to have sex more often, so let's figure out my orgasm. I'd like to up my average so it's closer to yours. Let's try a few new things to see if we can get me there."

Don't ask permission! Tell him that this is the new plan. Suggest he learns how to make a good margarita, the kind with fresh squeezed limes. Then tell him to do some research, too. (No, porn doesn't count.) Psych yourself up. Remind your brain how good it can feel when it's all over, when you're panting and relaxed, quiet and still, listening to the birds outside your window. The kids are fine, somewhere else.

Next step: make it happen. The same way you make all the other things happen. Find the damn time and then ask for what you need. Dim the lights and keep sipping that cocktail until you stop obsessing over all your perfect imperfections. Your body is a masterpiece of curves, soft and near.

Whisper, "Hey, try this."

Suggest some new things you've recently learned. Ask him to vary his approach, his rhythm and combinations. Position yourself where it's going to work best for you, even if it's missionary style. It's fine. He'll survive.

You know that incredible explosion your partner feels when they climax? You, too, deserve that every time. And if you figure out your mechanics so that you orgasm more, you'll want it more, too—it's a win-win! Use simple language, no apologetic vernacular, no dismissing or undervaluing the mission. Be the coach of your body. Be supportive of his efforts, but stay on him and guide him to victory.

In the same way you research tutors, coaches, and summer camps, it's high time you researched your own orgasm.

The goal is to be a wife and mother who still enjoys sex, reveling in the little adventure for what it is: a brief way to lose yourself, to giggle, and to maintain closeness that can feel extraordinarily amazing. Empower yourself to figure out what gets you there. Then, make time for it and let loose.

Sex is best when we own our desire for pleasure. So, claim your orgasm, my friend, and go get your fun.

🕐

V. C. Chickering is the author of Nookietown *and* Twisted Family Values.

Yes, But Not Now

WILLIAM DAMERON

When I walk into the bedroom wearing only a towel after my morning shower, Paul sits up in bed and asks, "Is there a show?"

After ten years of marriage, he still acts as though he has never seen my body, which is adorable, if not entirely believable. Part of this is habit, these things Paul says. The kids and I call them, Paul-isms. Like clockwork, they are as consistent as his sunny, good mood, which we have decided to find charming, if not entirely welcome—especially on a Monday morning.

"No," I mumble, "there is not a show."

He raises an eyebrow and cups a hand to his ear.

"Sorry," I say and then repeat another Paul-ism. "Yes, but not now."

We met a little over twelve years ago, on a Tuesday night in late November at the Cheesecake Factory in the Burlington Mall. I thought Paul was one of the most beautiful men I had ever seen. With his tall frame, handsome, symmetrical face and big toothy grin, he possesses an effortless charm that both women and men, especially gay ones—the lechers—admire.

At forty-three, I had been out of the closet for six months and could count on two fingers, maybe three depending upon your definition, my sexual experiences with men. Sitting across the table from Paul and his perfectly arranged face, all I wanted to do was kiss him. I lie. There was more I wanted to do, but I'm not that kind of writer.

I held out until our third date, having learned from the previous two, perhaps three, encounters with other men that appearing too hungry and desperate terrified them. Paul made dinner for me, a succulent pork roast in red wine sauce, and afterward by the fire we had "dessert." Three servings. Honestly, I thought he was out of my league and that he was too kind to say no. So, in my best Oliver Twist accent, I kept repeating, "Please sir, I want some more," which is what Paul wants now as he watches me getting dressed.

"Show me something," he mouths.

I zip up my pants.

After three months of dating, I accidentally let it slip. I was late for work because of a sleepover (really, you should assume everything I write that smacks of innuendo actually is). Heading toward the door, I kissed Paul and said it: "I love you."

When he replied that he loved me too, I thought he was too kind just to say, "Mm-kay," and when he agreed to marry me, I was not entirely convinced that he understood. But here I am a decade later, seldom having sex with my good-looking, good-natured husband.

This may come as a shock, but if you lock two half-naked, gay men in a bedroom, the end result is not always sex, though it used to be for us. As I pull on my shirt, I glance over at Paul and wonder, how did we get to this place?

Paul puts a finger to his tongue and pretends to tweak a nipple, inviting me to do the same.

I button up my shirt.

There are times when we are in public and the last golden rays of sunlight are caressing Paul's face and moments when we walk along a lonely stretch of New England beach that I think, yes, this. I see in his profile an irresistible, childlike wonder, and I want to reach out and clasp his hand or kiss his lips, but more than four decades of muscle memory are telling me Stop! Someone might see you—it's not safe; not now. So, all of my physical touch is funneled into the shadows. In this time and space and place, sandwiched between aging parents and adult children still at home, are mounting responsibilities, cooking, cleaning, reading emails, and writing to deadlines. There is only a small sliver of time for physical affection and splinters of that time are divvied up into sleep and sex. There are nights, becoming more frequent, when we roll from side to side, enjoying neither.

It was our youngest daughter, Celine, who is attuned to every tiny vibration of change in our household, who noticed—even before I did—that sunny-side Paul had become somewhat hard-boiled. When I walked into the kitchen one weekend morning she was sitting at the dining room table, a pile of college textbooks in front of her and a hand on her forehead. She looked up at me and said, "Dad seems out of sorts lately. Have I done something wrong?"

> In this time and space and place, sandwiched between aging parents and adult children still at home, are mounting responsibilities, cooking, cleaning, reading emails, and writing to deadlines.

I paused for a moment and concluded that at twenty-one years old, she could handle the truth.

"Oh no, no sweetie, he's not upset with you," I said, patting her hand. "Your father and I just haven't had sex in a while."

"Um," she replied, and then looked out the window. "Ew. Okay, but that's actually a relief. Is everything all right?"

"Oh, God, yes! We've just hit a dry spell."

"Again, a lot of information."

She stood up.

"That settles it. Ben and I are going to the movies tonight," she said, referring to her older brother. She flashed her eyebrows at me and said, "Rest up, sport, you've got a big night, tonight."

Walking to her bedroom, she paused and then slapped me on the rear end. "Go get him, tiger."

That night, I decided to spice things up by wearing my glasses, the readers with black plastic frames, during our lovemaking. I was going for the sexy, nerdy look. Afterward, my head resting in the crook of his arm, Paul turned to me, kissed my nose, and said, "What's with the grandpa look?"

Instead of getting angry, I started laughing uncontrollably, which reaffirmed my steadfast belief that I married exactly the right person, and as a bonus, we have a blended family with five beautifully irreverent, wonderful kids.

We're getting older, Paul and I, and with that comes creaking knees, spreading waistlines, and a decreasing libido, but looking over at Paul, all of him stretched out on the bed, I remembered that time by the fire. After that first night, while he was sleeping, I tiptoed to the bathroom and sobbed. It was too much, that unbearable voluminosity of emotions, consuming joy after a lifetime of denial.

Work can wait. I walk over to Paul while unbuttoning my shirt, and he places his smartphone down on the bed.

"I'm sorry," he says, smiling as he puts a hand to his ear and pulls out the earbud. "I'm on mute. Do you want something?"

"Yes," I say, cupping my hand around his perfect face—yes, dear husband, I do. "But not now."

🕐

Bill Dameron is an award-winning blogger, essayist, and the author of The Lie: A Memoir of Two Marriages, Catfishing & Coming Out.

How to Have Sex with a Germaphobe

CLAIRE GIBSON

scrubbed my classroom surfaces with Lysol wipes. I used hand sanitizer religiously. And still, during my first semester as a middle school teacher, I caught a nasty virus.

Around the same time that I started teaching, I fell in love with Patrick, a Nashville native with a thick red beard, freckles, and a penchant for plaid shirts. Those first few months, our dates often included a bottle of wine and a stack of papers to grade. His red pen was swift, likely because he was doing the math: the sooner the papers were graded, the sooner we could start making out. And make out we did. A lot.

It was a stressful year: a student threw a dictionary at my head. A colleague cornered me in my own classroom to shout me down for being insensitive. During those months, Patrick's kindness and help (and yes, his hot bod) bolstered my courage to face each new challenge. When I struggled to fall asleep, he'd stay by my side a bit longer, hold me close, and whisper in my ear, "Rest, love. Just rest."

Perhaps that's why I fell so hard, and why, only five months in, I said yes to his marriage proposal. Patrick's steady, calming presence had become an essential ingredient in my emotional stability. Though I'd dated plenty of men, there was something different about Patrick. My experience of physical intimacy in the past had always felt like an act of subtraction. But kissing Patrick felt like an act of multiplication. We were young and in love. And so we made out, oblivious to the germs passing from the students to the teacher to her fiancée.

A few days after he proposed, Patrick got a sore throat. While we drove to Georgia to be with my family, he called his doctor and begged for a prescription to calm his irritated lungs. The entire Christmas break, while I was high on the adrenaline of new love and wedding plans, he was high on cough syrup and ibuprofen. We kissed and canoodled through it all, germs be damned. Not wanting to ruin my time with family, Patrick pretended he was well.

We entwine our bodies and believe in our souls and connect at a distance that the government will never control.

Only now, ten years into our marriage, do I realize what a feat of love that must have required.

Though he hid it well during our short engagement, my husband is a bona fide germaphobe. He elbow-bumps like a champ. He washes his hands until they're so dry they crack. At work events, if a stranger offers his (potentially germ-infested) business card, my husband snaps a photo of the contact info with his iPhone, and then puts his hands in his pockets and says he doesn't like clutter.

Throughout our marriage, Patrick has taught me the art of social distancing. Only, before this coronavirus outbreak, I simply thought he was being rude. For example, earlier this winter I had a runny nose and itchy throat. Properly medicated (thank you, Dayquil), I grabbed my purse and prepared to leave the house for work. On the way out, I leaned in to kiss Patrick goodbye, only to feel him pull his head back slightly, purse his lips together, and wince. Properly rejected, I went from loving to completely pissed off in a nanosecond.

"What the heck?" I snapped.

"I don't want to get sick," he explained.

"You could at least hug me," I huffed. "You don't have to treat me like a leper."

"I'm just playing it safe. We both don't have to get sick."

This is a common argument—one that gets replayed every flu season without fail. Me, pooh-poohing the natural laws of communicable diseases, and my husband, holding strong so that at least one of us is well enough to parent our two young children. For years, I've held the pessimistic mindset that if I get sick, we're all going to get sick. Patrick takes a different tack. If one of us gets sick, he goes into battle mode, ready to hole himself away to ward off the domino effect. Forget sex; if one of us is sick, we usually end up sleeping in separate beds. I stew, feeling rejected. Patrick shrugs, knowing he is ultimately helping our family get better faster.

For years I raged against his precautions. And then, a new, deadly disease emerged on the face of the globe—one so contagious, it had the potential to infect hundreds of thousands of people, and might just shut down the entire world economy. In the weeks before the United States finally understood what it was up against with COVID-19, I tentatively began asking Patrick about his strategies to avoid germs. He encouraged me to change my hand-washing habits (as in, do it more, Claire). When I began to feel worried—about our friends in the restaurant industry, about my friend who owns a home-cleaning business that will likely go under, about my parents who refuse to believe that the virus is real—his still, calm voice continues to offer reassurance.

It's an act of resistance against the forces of evil that will try to pull us apart . . . It's a silent shout that screams, "Hell no. Heaven yes."

For now, we are both well. We are practicing social distancing from our dear neighbors and friends in Nashville, many of whom are still reeling from a tornado that passed through three weeks ago. And so at night, he reaches for me. He caresses my shoulder. I kiss his mouth. He doesn't pull back. We entwine our bodies and believe in our souls and connect at a distance that the government will never control.

At a marriage conference several years ago, the speaker explained that sex is an act of outrageous hope. It's an act of resistance against the forces of evil that will try to pull us apart. It is a moment of total presence, of silence, of belief that life and pleasure and ecstasy can still exist in the midst of chaos. It's a silent shout that screams, "Hell no. Heaven yes."

In the afterglow, my husband whispers in my ear.

"Rest, love. Just rest."

His steady, calming influence is more important now than ever. And if one of us gets sick? Patrick has a plan. He's ready to quarantine himself or provide so that I could do the same. We don't both have to get sick, he reminds me. He's ready to ensure that our family stays safe. Is there anything sexier than that?

Claire Gibson is the author of Beyond the Point, *which is currently in development with a major Hollywood studio.*

What My Mother Taught Me about Sex

CAITLIN MULLEN

Our conversation lasted ten minutes, but in my mind it stretched hours.

was sure my mom wouldn't know what hit her.

"I have something to tell you," I said. I was seven years old and couldn't help but gloat about what I had learned that afternoon. I felt so adult—so brimming with classified knowledge—I had to blurt it out.

"What's that?" she asked. Distracted, my mother glanced over her shoulder at me, then quickly returned to preparing dinner.

"Jamie told me all about sex."

I expected my mother to pivot, mouth agape. Instead, she turned around slowly and eyed me with a smile playing at the corners of her lips.

"Oh yeah?" she said. There was a knowing sound to her voice.

It took me nearly a decade to realize that my mother had seen this coming from a mile away. My friend Jamie was two years older than me and only played with me because the power balance always fell in her favor. A quiet and obedient playmate, I lived across the street and blindly believed anything Jamie told me, hanging on her every word.

Jamie relished her natural superiority. Earlier that year, my play-mate had convinced me that it was imperative for us to wear her mom's panty liners in our underwear. In middle school, it was Jamie who introduced me to porn, fanning through a stack of Playboys that her dad kept underneath his side of the bed. The first time she shaved her legs, she imme-diately ran over to my house and ordered me to stroke her hairless shins. This was the kind of friend she was—older, wiser, ready to school me in whatever new milestone she had reached.

To me, sex was a vague and furtive adult activity, something that lurked beneath the surface.

No wonder my mother wasn't surprised.

"What exactly did Jamie tell you?" my mom asked. While she knew Jamie was that friend, she also knew that Jamie likely didn't have the full story.

I squirmed in my chair, then looked away, feeling certain that I'd overplayed my hand. What had Jamie told me, exactly? I combed through my memory of the play date. With a knowing smile, Jamie had stripped off Barbie and Ken's clothes and mashed their bodies together with a violence I now assume was meant to stand-in for passion.

She'd said, "They're going to have sex."

I nodded, pretending to know what she meant.

To me, sex was a vague and furtive adult activity, something that lurked beneath the surface. There were glimpses of this hidden real-ity everywhere I looked. In the movies my parents wouldn't let me watch. In magazine advertisements, where women wore lingerie in order to sell liquor or lotion or cruise ship vacations. In the sitcom jokes that flew over my head. In the song lyrics I belted out but didn't fully understand.

My mom interpreted my hesitation correctly, sighed, and pulled out a chair.

"Okay," she said. "I'm going to tell you what you need to know."

With unsparing and anatomically correct detail, my mother revealed to me what happened when two people had sex. She spoke about body parts inserted into other body parts, about sperm and eggs. I thought for a moment about what Ken and Barbie looked like underneath their clothes. The dolls, with those featureless, neutered spaces between their legs, were not at all up to the task of demonstrating the things my mother had just spoken about. Everything about Jamie's Barbie tutorial fell remarkably short in depicting the truth my mother was now imparting to me.

My mother was my safe place, even when I felt like my world had been shattered.

My mother's sex talk probably lasted ten minutes, but in my mind it stretched hours, my face turning a deeper shade of red with every passing second. I was simultaneously trying to process the facts as she was laying them out while also coming to terms with just how quickly I had gone from feeling adult and worldly to clueless and chagrined.

"Of course," my mom said, as she got up from the table, "people also do it for fun. Including me and your dad."

The mention of my parents having sex made me bury my face in my hands. If I hadn't been prepared to learn the real mechanics of sex, I certainly hadn't been prepared to picture my parents doing it either. And fun? I don't know what I was thinking when Jamie gave me the Barbie demonstration, other than sex was something adults were compelled to do the same way they seemed mysteriously compelled to vacuum the floor of the car.

"If you have questions, you know you can ask me, right?"

I managed a meek nod. And with that, my mother patted my hand and went back to making dinner as though nothing had happened at all.

My initial reaction was shock, but later I thought of things a little differently. By leading a frank, unashamed discussion about sex, my mother also taught me that she would be there for other difficult conversations throughout my life. She taught me that honesty—especially when it is uncomfortable—is a way to demonstrate love. Jamie told me about sex so that she could revel in feeling more powerful, more sophisticated than me. But my mom, with her straight-faced descriptions, told me for the opposite reason: so that I might feel armed by the knowledge, empowered by it.

Jamie and I drifted apart after middle school. As she fell into a crowd of her same-age peers, I grew more preoccupied with books and schoolwork. But my mother and I would have years of conversations at that same kitchen table. Difficult conversations and sad ones, such as how to deal with my first real breakup and deciding when to go back to college after my father died. Each time, my mother was my safe place, even when I felt like my world had been shattered. Each time, I came away with the same feeling as I did that day my mom told me the truth about sex. That no matter what I had gone out in the world to experience for myself, I could always come back to her to help me close the gap between what I knew and what I still needed to learn.

🕐

Caitlin Mullen is the debut author of the novel Please See Us.

Don't Crush My Butterflies

ZIBBY OWENS

I was almost forty years old, but I felt like a teenager.

was the only grown-up angling to get more fire on my marshmallow. Little kids shoved me out of the way as we jousted with our extra-long bamboo sticks for the perfect roasting position. It was my first vacation without kids since I'd had kids, and there I was, around a firepit in Puerto Rico, packed in with everyone else's.

I'd recently separated from my husband and had fallen in love with the man who I would end up remarrying. Kyle and I were in the butterfly stage of our love affair: We couldn't stand to be apart. When we were together, we were constantly touching, swooning, smooching, and staring into each other's eyes. I was almost forty years old then, but I felt like a teenager. My body responded to Kyle's in such a physical way: heart fluttering when I saw him, cheeks blushing, tummy warm, drawn into his arms like a magnet.

This was our first big trip together. My first Christmas break week without the kids. We walked arm in arm through the winding security line, stopping to kiss, hug, and touch. The disgruntled passport officer looked at us and snapped, "Looks like someone's in love." We didn't need anything external to keep us occupied on the plane. We talked and laughed the whole way. The plastic barrier between our seats felt insurmountable and when the seatbelt sign dinged off, I got up and just snuggled into his lap.

"You know this stage is going to end, right?" I told him. He looked at me like I was crazy.

"Don't crush my butterflies," he said. "I'll always have them!" I hoped he was right, but having fallen in and out of love many times, I wasn't optimistic about that early stage lingering. I missed it while I was still in it.

At the resort that week, I alternated between realities. I waffled between the extreme sadness, anguish, and physical pain at being so far apart from my kids, who felt like an extension of my soul; and elation, electric attraction, and excitement at being with Kyle. Before meeting him, I realized a part of myself was dead. The fire inside me, what made me me, had been stamped out after a decade of decline. I'd felt like the inside of an old-fashioned barbecue grill long after dinner, a smoking pit of burnt charcoal briquettes, white with traces of fire, cracking at the edges, black smoke rising. Done.

"You know this stage is going to end, right?" I told him. He looked at me like I was crazy. "Don't crush my butterflies," he said. "I'll always have them!"

Now, suddenly, I was in full blaze, flames flying over the lid of the grill, dancing in the dark. Alive again. And yet, torn apart from the loves of my life for a week that felt endless, I would cry at random times, moon over pictures of them, and mourn as I felt the rope connecting me to them pulling and pulling. It felt familiar, like grief. But then I would shape-shift into a sex-starved adolescent, smoking with sensation as I got to know my new love.

That night when I saw the crowd forming around the resort's firepit, I raced over. I was there not to help my four kids make s'mores, but because I loved s'mores myself and wanted to make them. For me.

Kyle and I were laughing and flirting as we roasted the puffy white confections. An exhausted, downcast mother lording over her sugar-packed kids on the other side of the firepit looked at us, sighed, and said, "What I wouldn't give for just one minute of that feeling again."

I think about that mother every day.

On so many days, I am that mother. And for so long, I was her every day. I had lost hope. I had relegated those emotions to the past while stuck in the sands of twenty-four/seven parenthood. But then, suddenly, I was reborn.

The fire inside me, what made me me, had been stamped out after a decade of decline. I'd felt like the inside of an old-fashioned barbecue grill long after dinner, a smoking pit of burnt charcoal briquettes . . .

"I have four kids!" I told her. "I'm the same as you! I felt the same way. But it can happen! It can!" She shook her head, resigned to her fate. We kept chatting over the fire. My new self was confronted with a version of my old self. I touched her arm and smiled as I walked away. I watched her with her family over the next week, waving as we crossed paths.

It has been almost five years since that trip. Everything has changed. Puerto Rico was crushed in a massive hurricane. The pandemic wreaked havoc across the globe. Travel is barely possible. I'm ensconced in my home with my four kids and Kyle, now my husband of three years.

The butterflies still flutter around us, but they've been tempered by world events, stress, ups and downs, losses, illnesses, and other struggles that life brings. The other night, as I was racing around upstairs, exhausted, folding laundry and trying to get my two teenagers and two little guys to bed, I glanced out back and saw Kyle and a friend of ours roasting marshmallows at our outdoor fireplace. I felt a stab of longing. Had I become that exhausted, resigned mom again?

As I put tiny tank tops away inside my daughter's closet, Kyle came bounding in, proudly offering up a s'more he had made just for me. I couldn't even eat it.

"I can't now," I said. "I'm still doing laundry and have to get the kids to bed and . . ."

"But I made it perfectly, just the way you like it!" he said. I just shook my head. He walked out, dejected, taking the s'more with him.

I immediately regretted how I'd handled it. Why hadn't I let myself enjoy the treat? Why couldn't I have stopped the chaos for a minute and let my own needs be met? Why hadn't I let my husband make me happy, something that would have made him feel satisfied and proud?

I found the s'more on my bedside table later as I climbed into bed, and left it beside me uneaten. It sat there all night as the two of us slept.

The next morning when I saw it, I felt overcome by remorse. I rolled over and snuggled in with Kyle while he slept. Why had I handled things so badly? I got up and tossed the s'more into the garbage, then covered it up with tissues so he wouldn't see.

I miss those butterflies. I know they're still fluttering around us. And I know I'm the one who doesn't always stop to see them. But I know they're there, dancing overhead.

🕐

Zibby Owens is a writer and mother of four in New York City. She is a literary advocate and the creator and host of the award-winning literary podcast Moms Don't Have Time to Read Books. *She runs a literary salon with author events, a virtual book club, and a daily* Z-IGTV *live author interview series.*

Now's Not the Time
WENDY WALKER

Recently, I was at a man's house for a date. We'd been together for a few months. His house was empty. My house had just one teenager who was probably psyched that I was out of his hair for the night. As we sat on the couch searching for something to watch, having together time, building our relationship so it wouldn't die from lack of oxygen, I felt a powerful desire to go home. Yes, my son would ignore me. Yes, he would spend the night FaceTiming his girlfriend while I watched Netflix in the next room. Still, he would know I was there, and I could not stop my feet from walking out the door.

I went home. The relationship ended. And I had an epiphany.

I have felt societal pressure to have a man in my life since I was a young girl. If I didn't have one, then finding one was on my list of things to do. Sometimes at the very bottom, sometimes at the top, it was always there. On The List. Even after my divorce, when I was struggling to rebuild my life, take care of children, navigate a new career, I saw it back there. Near the top. In bold. In red ink. In flashing neon lights. And so, like most items on The List, I tended to this item with calculated diligence. Online dating, blind dates, matchmaking services, compromises, self-doubt, and a constant degradation of my standards. So he lives in his mother's basement—maybe it's just a rough patch?

After a few painful years, I was very fortunate to meet a wonderful man, and I have no doubt that under different circumstances we would have shared an incredible life together. Violins, please. But wait . . . together we had six children, two jobs, and no path forward to merge our families. What we loved most about each other was the very thing that did us in—our children were at the top of our lists.

I have felt societal pressure to have a man in my life since I was a young girl.

I was devastated but, rather than throw in the towel, I became more determined than ever to find a solution.

I decided to move this line item to the top of The List, and found a man ready to blend his family with mine. All in. One house. This ended with near-disastrous results. I moved back into my old house three months later and also moved the line item back to where it belonged. Below my children, my career, and my stable home.

Fast-forward three more years to the man and the couch. As kind and fun as he was, I felt something different when I walked out the door. Relief. It was then that the epiphany came.

It came to me like a perfect plot twist. As most writers well know, sometimes the best twist comes after diving deeper into the minutiae of the original premise. But other times, you have to zoom out and look at all of the assumptions that you made when you started the plot to begin with. Maybe the victim doesn't die! Suddenly, a whole new story can be written.

So rather than dive back in to attack this line item of finding a man, I zoomed out and asked the broader question of whether this item had to be on The List at all. At this stage of my life, I had everything that I needed to be happy. Three great children who were almost launched into the world. A supportive family. Two handfuls of very close friends. And a hard-won career which I not only enjoyed but which had introduced me to a community of smart, supportive, and hilariously irreverent people. I had friendship, plans every Saturday night, financial security, deep satisfaction from all that I had accomplished, the ability to give back to others, and a home for my family that I had created and loved beyond measure.

For the first time in my life, I took this item off The List. And something wonderful happened. I began to see myself through a completely different lens.

I stopped caring about how many likes I had on an app or second glances I caught from across a room, but rather what I wanted to accomplish each day for myself, for my career, for my family.

I started to feel about finding a man the way I feel when I walk past items at the grocery store that I don't need that week. Complete indifference. And with that indifference came a freedom that I had never experienced before. I used that freedom to write two novels, deepen my friendships, tend to my children with heightened mindfulness, and—as a nice bonus—to get into the best physical shape I have been in since my years as a competitive figure skater.

The time will soon come when all of my children are off doing their own things and I'll be grateful if I get a phone call once a week. A day will come when I have more time to give and less to lose by giving it. Then, I'll know that it's the right time to add this item back to The List. And when that happens, I will do so with careful intent on finding not just time for a man, but a lasting relationship of substance that will add joy to my life, and allow me to add joy to someone else's.

> I started to feel about finding a man the way I feel when I walk past items at the grocery store that I don't need that week. Complete indifference.

🕐

Wendy Walker is the author of thrillers The Night Before *and* Don't Look For Me. *A former attorney specializing in family law, her novels include* Emma in the Night *and* All Is Not Forgotten.

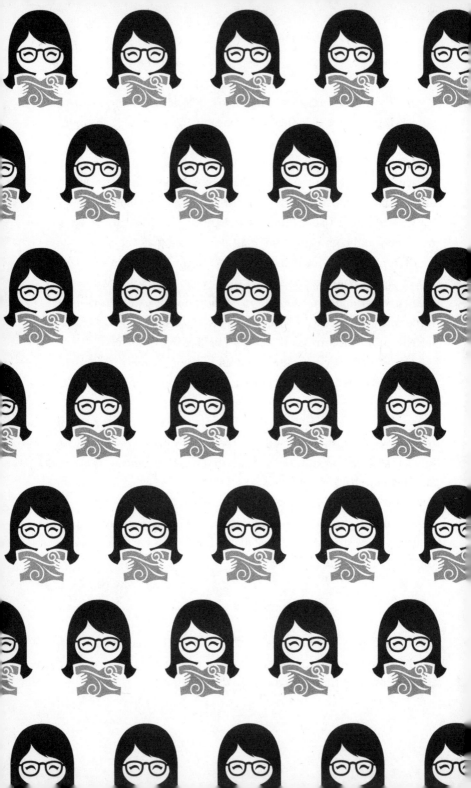

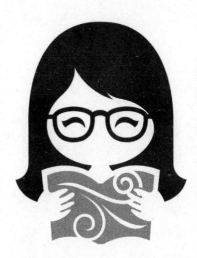

MOMS
DON'T HAVE
TIME TO
BREATHE

Moms Don't Have Time to Cry
LIZ ASTROF

Before kids, shedding tears was my prerogative.

I really needed to cry.

I had just gotten news of a death: not a death related to me, but rather, the death of a friend's mother. I had only met her once, so normally I wouldn't have cried over this news, but my friend and her mother had a closeness that my own mother and I never shared, which triggered me. This upsetting news was compounded by the fact that my son's principal told me he wasn't picking up on social cues, and the thought of him being rejected by his peers broke my heart—I still hadn't gotten around to crying about that. Earlier that week, I'd met a US Navy veteran who had rescued an older dog from death row at the pound. I told him he was a hero for saving the dog's life, but he explained that after serving in Afghanistan and suffering from PTSD, that the dog had actually saved him. The dog saved him! So, there were also some happy tears still waiting to be shed.

Moral of the story: I couldn't cry about any of these things at the appropriate times, because I have children. Between feeding them, scheduling playdates, doctor visits, helping with homework, filling out field trip forms, buying new shoes (why do their feet grow so fast?!), drying their tears, and the millions of other "Mom, can you . . ." and "Mom, I need . . ." moments that pop up incessantly filling any gaps of time that might have otherwise been considered free, I don't have time to cry. Most moms don't.

It's not easy to satisfy our innate need to keep it all together for the kids at times when the pull to feel emotion—to be human—feels just as compelling. Eventually, the emotion will have to come out, like a splinter, or the truth. We just have to wait for the perfect opportunity to present itself.

The world was my crying oyster.

Once my kids are tucked into bed, I am free to lose my shit. Unfortunately, by the time I do all of the other things that I put off doing (like talking to my husband, and every so often, having sex with him so we don't become estranged), I have hardly enough time to rewatch the first ten minutes of whatever Netflix show everyone is bingeing, before I pass out. The argument could be made for crying during sex. However, that's when I make my shopping lists. (I can only multitask so much.)

Before I had kids, I unknowingly took a lot of little things for granted, like the value of the emotional release that accompanies the tears-pouring-down-your-face, runny-nose, use your sleeve as a tissue because you had no idea it was going to be that kind of cry, cry. Back then, I could cry whenever the urge arose: on the subway, on the street, in a cab, in a bar, in a bathroom, on my way home. I could cry at home. And when I did cry at home, I didn't have to hide. I could walk from room to room just . . . crying. I could also cry about one thing at a time. I didn't have to do my crying in bulk, like I do now.

Once my kids are tucked into bed, I am free to lose my shit.

The world was my crying oyster.

The shower has always been a great place for me to cry. These days, though, I'm always in such a rush that my showers are more of a three-in-one body wash/shampoo/conditioner situation with no time to access true emotion. On top of that, I'm constantly being interrupted by the "urgent" needs of my children. Even if I am so bold as to lock the bathroom door, I have to brace myself for the pounding and screaming that will inevitably ensue—noise that can easily pierce the barrier of any running shower, regardless of how strong the pressure. Even when they're not pounding on the door, I'm waiting for them to pound on the door. The same goes for my closet, or any room with a dead bolt on the door.

Luckily, as a working mother, I do have some time to cry—like in traffic during my commute. One morning, I got into my car and before I could even get to my iTunes "Crying Mix" playlist featuring R.E.M's "Everybody Hurts" and Elton John's "Candle in the Wind" (I mean, why not?), I turned on the car and a bouncy song erupted from the speakers. Of course, I had to sing along. Once the song ended, my crying mood was gone, but I was determined. I needed the release that badly.

The argument could be made for crying during sex. However, that's when I make my shopping lists. (I can only multitask so much.)

Just as the lump was beginning to return to my throat, my phone rang. I didn't recognize the number, so I let it go straight to voice-mail. But then I wondered who it was and what they wanted. It could have been a notice about a late payment on a bill. Or the pharmacy calling to say that my Xanax prescription was ready. (Or worse, not ready.) The caller didn't leave a voice mail, but somehow the brief interruption in my scheduled crying time ruined it for me.

That weekend, when my cry was way, way past due, I took my kids to see *Toy Story 3*. Toward the end, happy tears sprung to my eyes. It was finally time for my long-overdue cry session! But then my son, seven years old at the time, turned to me, head tilted, a concerned look upon his face, and said, "I have to go number two."

I had to call it off.

I had all but given up, but then later that evening I was in the kitchen making stir-fry and I sliced into a particularly potent onion. Before I could finish peeling it, my nose was burning and tears were streaming from my eyes. Next thing I knew, I wasn't just crying onion tears. I was crying real tears. With my back to my kids, I wept. I wept about all of the things I needed to cry about, and other things that I had forgotten about.

It was guttural. It was ugly. It was glorious. And I had earned it.

We all ate my tears for dinner. And it tasted like relief.

Liz Astrof is an award-winning executive producer and sitcom writer. She is the author of Don't Wait Up: Confessions of a Stay-at-Work Mom.

The Life-Changing Magic of Letting Go

JEANNE McWILLIAMS BLASBERG

A midlife reckoning with my stuff.

I once took a class in the art of memoir where the assignment was to write about an object and its meaning. I bristled at the prompt. Objects are only objects, I told myself, and imbuing them with meaning was materialistic and shallow. It was akin to idolatry, which is against my religion, by the way. Besides, I was a mom trying to keep up with the stream of macaroni art, woodshop creations, and papier-mâché coming through the door.

Eschewing sentimentality, I had been known to sweep entire tabletops of clutter into garbage bags. Oh sure, I'd hang my children's masterpieces on the refrigerator for the requisite number of weeks, but they'd eventually get sent to the circular file . . . wink wink.

In hindsight, I've realized that curation is a luxury for late middle-age, when the kids are out of the house and the mind is quiet. In my thirties and forties I'd vacillate between two extremes, either going on a rampage of throwing things away or pasting mementos from obvious milestones into albums. Now in my fifties, I fear I memorialized the wrong things and tossed the right ones. What I wouldn't give for more samples of my kids' poetry or handwriting. I wish I had recorded the peal of their laughter, their voices in the back seat of the car, the knock-knock jokes, the potty humor.

In addition to albums of meaningless certificates and a smattering of Little League trophies, I've held on to practical items, furnishings I thought might make their transition to adulthood easier (maybe something of me they would want to take with them?). But no matter how often I suggest shipping a useful household appliance to one of our three adult children (a knife sharpener!), the answer is always the same, "It's okay, Mom, I'm all set."

Now in my fifties, I fear I memorialized the wrong things and tossed the right ones. What I wouldn't give for more samples of my kids' poetry or handwriting.

What we decide to hold on to is foremost on my mind as my husband and I move his ninety-two-year-old father out of his apartment. Despite all the work to be done, I find myself lingering among his decades-old artifacts, suddenly filled with compassion for the hoarding nature I was once so quick to criticize. He has kept yellowed envelopes containing locks of hair and God-awful pottery paperweights. It's becoming clear we humans cling to things as a way of holding on to the past, fearing memories will disappear if we let go of the objects that trigger them.

Coincidentally, as I've been ruminating on "object worship," what to keep and what must go, my daily meditation from Melody Beattie's *Journey to the Heart* was this:

> [Fill] your life and your world with the colors, textures, scents, and objects that are beautiful to you, that have meaning to you. . . . Carefully and thoughtfully choose the items you place in your home. Objects have energy, when we obtain them, and the energy and meaning we attribute to them. . . . they tell a story all day long.

Turns out my memoir teacher was the wise one after all.

While our friends are shedding family homes and downsizing, I'm caught between generations, in a weird state of limbo, the steward of family treasures that I don't necessarily have a link to, but nonetheless, feel responsible for. The thing is, I want to be less like the custodian of a family museum and more like Beattie: the curator of my life's surroundings.

I asked Ali Wenzke, author of *The Art of Happy Moving*, for help. She reinforced what I have begun to sense. "As we get older," she told me, "we begin to accumulate generations' worth of items from our parents and from our children. Keep the items that mean the most to you or that meant the most to your parents, but let go of the rest. They would want you to move forward and to not be encumbered by the past. You can hold your loved ones in your memory without being surrounded by their belongings."

Besides listening to Ali, I should take a lesson from my children who so deftly resist the gifts I try to bequeath. As always, I suspect my current struggle goes back to a childhood wound (doesn't it always?). You see, when I left California for Massachusetts to attend college eons ago, my parents also moved to Texas and discarded all I'd left in my room, the detritus of my life to that point. They were mostly silly objects, I know, in their eyes not worth shipping, but what stung was the fact that I never gave my permission or had a chance to say goodbye.

Despite having craved a measure of sentimentality from my own parents, I grew up to mock it in others. I actually snickered upon learning my husband's parents had saved all his report cards. Now, in midlife, I get it.

The irony is that despite having craved a measure of sentimentality from my own parents, I grew up to mock it in others. I actually snickered upon learning my husband's parents had saved all his report cards. Now, in midlife, I get it.

They say being self-aware is the first step toward recovery. I think that's why I was fascinated by Marie Kondo early on, and found her advice to assess an object's ability to "spark joy" illuminating. Incidentally, while perusing a bookstore this past weekend, I stumbled upon a book called *The Gentle Art of Swedish Death Cleaning* by Margareta Magnusson. It describes a Swedish phenomenon called *döstädning*, whereby you cull your possessions so your loved ones don't have to do it after you pass. I was like: okay, Universe, I hear you!

These days, I'm trying to channel my younger self, the one who delighted in recycling, donating, and dropping full trash bags on the curb while being mindful of the setting I aim to create. I may not have had the time or the foresight to curate before, but I'm adopting an intentional collector's eye going forward. And I'm finding *döstädning* to be like any practice—writing, meditation, yoga—doing a little every day makes a big difference.

Jeanne McWilliams Blasberg is a travel writer and author of the novels Eden *and* The Nine.

My Mother and Me:
An Unrequited Love Story

DEBORAH BURNS

She always seemed to be forever beyond my grasp.

Breathing was difficult when I was a child. It wasn't asthma, or a wheeze, or any other respiratory ailment. Quite simply, there was no air left in the room for me; my mother had inhaled it all.

I was the only child of a preternaturally beautiful, larger-than-life mother, and the spell that she cast upon me (and everyone else) remains vivid twenty-five years after her death. I worshipped her—idolized her, really—and merrily danced around the pedestal of a goddess no mere mortal like myself could ever hope to become. When she was alive, I was always in chasing mode, a longing pursuit of something fleeting. She seemed to forever be just beyond my grasp, and her elusiveness stoked my deepest, darkest fear: my mother doesn't really love me.

"You look nothing like your mother, Debbie." This oft-repeated line haunted my childhood, especially because I wanted nothing more than to embody my mother's movie star gorgeousness.

My inner voice taunted me: If only I looked more like her, maybe she would be with me more. The appeal of my own soulful brown eyes versus her piercing blues; of my bittersweet chocolate hair versus her seductive red mane didn't matter much then. How easily love and beauty can get tangled for a sensitive child trying to make sense of the way things were. Even if I had heard of narcissism then, I was far too young to understand it.

Once, decked out in a dazzling lime-green suit with a silver fox fur collar, my mother and I went to the Central Park Zoo. An enormous gorilla soon caught sight of her and began to wildly pace and pant and issue the most guttural, rolling grunts as he pulled at his bars in a frenzy. Onlookers cheered as she walked by his cage again and again. I stood back as this primal scene unfolded, a silent witness to the undeniable truth of my mother's power.

My fears were fed by my mother's outside-the-lines unconventionality. Her abandonment of domesticity—and day-to-day mothering—went completely against the grain of the conservative 1950s. Defying her era's constraints, my mother designed a life that suited her needs. She planted her two spinster sisters-in-law—my short, plump, fairy godmother aunts—into our tiny Queens apartment and quickly turned my daily care over to them. She fully owned her rebel persona, dismissing fussing schoolyard moms who knitted sweaters and made heart-shaped sandwiches. Instead, my mother blew in and out like a VIP guest walking the red carpet between her bedroom and the front door.

"My darling girl! How are you today? Come! Follow me and help me change."

As I scampered alongside in that tight squeeze of an apartment, I wondered what other excitement had flushed her cheeks.

"Why are your bangs so short?"

Suddenly under her gaze, I could tell my mother was displeased.

"Lilly," she called out to the aunt responsible for my grooming. "Did you cut her hair with a bowl around her head?"

"It's humid today, so it curled up a bit," Lilly responded, eyes down.

"We all know her hair does that," my mother pronounced. "You have to take that into account."

Ahead of her time, she was the only mother in our circle who worked. In truth, she didn't want to and hated the office manager ordinariness, but our teetering finances required her income. She made up for her disappointment, however, by going out four to five nights each week with admirers who jockeyed for their spot in her orbit. It was an admirable independence a generation ago that would probably be applauded by many women today. But it left a wake of not feeling like her priority.

Back then, I dreamed that I would one day be the perfect mother. Where she was absent and removed from my day-to-day, I vowed to be present and in the weeds. My children would feel fully loved and get every single ounce of attention they deserved.

I soon became part of the boomer generation of women who had careers en masse and bought into the myth of "having it all." But after I married and birthed the first of my trio, a tug-of-war began as I struggled to balance my budding magazine career with the nurturing mother I wanted to become.

When my eldest was two, I chased a flexible schedule and crafted a (then unheard-of) three-day workweek. That schedule lasted for twelve years, and I kept my promise to parent differently. When I was home, I tended to mundane (but meaning-ful) tasks, to every bruise and ballet class, every tear and triumph.

> I dreamed that I would one day be the perfect mother. Where she was absent and removed from my day-to-day, I vowed to be present and in the weeds.

But as the years went on, work beckoned, and when my youngest was eight, I found myself thirty thousand feet in the air more often than I had ever imagined. I was struck with a new kind of breathlessness. Even though I had started with clear intentions, I'd slowly evolved into someone who was as absent as my mother was. That notion threatened me to the core.

These days, it's so much easier to view my lifelong conundrum from on high. And the good news? Every hand-wringing worry I ever had was for naught. If you injected any of my three adult children with truth serum and asked, "Does your mother love you?" they'd laugh.

And for that, I have my mother to thank. Her detachment spurred me toward connection with my own children. Her distance inspired me to dive deeper, even when it stretched me to the brink.

🕐

Deborah Burns is media consultant, speaker, and author of the memoir Saturday's Child: A Daughter's Memoir.

White Noise

LEA CARPENTER

Some thoughts on loss.

I opened Instagram this morning to find a post from a close friend whose father died yesterday. Here were the images she had chosen: her father holding her and her sisters on his lap (gentle); her father as a young man in swim trunks (handsome); her father by her side on her wedding day (traditional). She wrote about how he was her rock, how he quoted poetry, and also how he knew success in life didn't come from money or power. The post wasn't about her pain, though she must have woken up in pain. The post was about gratitude.

It takes a long time to get to gratitude in my experience. It takes a long time to even get to grief. In my experience the first phase of loss isn't grief at all—it's shock. It's white noise. All you really want in the hours after loss is to, as Auden put it, "stop all the clocks."

My father died before Instagram. I remember those early days as ones of retreating into a very small cell of family. There was lots of cooking and denial. Rage came later. I have written so much about my father since he died that it's almost embarrassing. What am I hoping to achieve? I wrote my first novel about him. On the surface, the story was about a mother whose son goes missing, but I was channeling my experience of a father who had, it felt, gone missing, too. I kept thinking I could bring him back by writing about him, that maybe the act of telling, and retelling who he was would open a path for his return. Magical thinking—right.

In my experience, magical thinking can become an addiction.

As I wrote about the anger my character felt about her son, I was describing my own anger, even though I didn't know it at the time.

In my experience the first phase of loss isn't grief at all—it's shock. It's white noise.

Of course writing didn't bring him back. My second novel was about a girl who loses her father too soon. I had done it again. I had tried to take my loss and reverse it on the page. Maybe one day my boys will read these books, I thought, and understand something they can't by looking at a photograph.

I helped my son with his book report on Operation Market Garden, an Allied airborne assault against the Germans. "It was the largest airborne assault, like, ever," my son explained, carefully articulating the word "assault," assuming that word might be foreign to me. He showed me maps that Churchill and Roosevelt had used. My son doesn't know that my father planned and executed "operations," too, though it didn't feel like the right moment to get into it. My father to my boys is an idea, a chimera. Would it matter to them that he had wanted to be a pilot? Would it matter that, due to poor eyesight, he instead was sent to do something different, something that might be described as "dangerous"? Dangerous is a word my boys love; if you're twelve, dangerous is slang for cool.

Before wanting to be a pilot, my father had wanted to be a cowboy. Early on in his time in the military he wrote to his mother that, "so far, I believe I am going to like my new job tremendously, all of it is outdoors, and not unlike my Western experiences. Couldn't help remembering the days when my idea of a perfect life was to ride through the hills packing a .45 and carrying a carbine, and now I'm paid to do it."

My father spent the last decade of his life working to overturn the mandatory-minimum sentencing laws in his home state, Delaware. When, eventually, the governor signed a bill into law ensuring the end of the "man mins," it was nicknamed "Ned's Bill" after my father. My mother and I went to the courthouse and sat at an enormous oblong table as the governor spoke about the importance of these laws and their place in a larger, urgent, national challenge: criminal justice reform, and a path to better race relations. That larger challenge was what my father felt was the critical issue facing this country.

Two days before he died, I received a letter, FedEx. I was on my way to the train station because my mother had called and said, "it's time," which meant, time to come home. Which meant, he's dying. I stood in the small hallway of my building and read the letter, which detailed why my father had decided I was the child to carry on his work with the "man-mins." Before I had finished reading it, my phone rang. It was my brother, calling to tell me he had received a letter, FedEx, from our father, and that his letter explained why he was the child to carry on the work.

I never saw my father rageful, but he must have had anger at times. He tried to channel his anger into action.

Had my father written the exact same letter to all of his children? I never found out the answer. Soon I was on the train, then by his bed, and then my baby boy was crying and I was holding my sister's hand and then he was gone. Later someone said, "no one will ever love you like he did," an idea at the time that I received as an insult. Later, I understood it as a very high compliment.

Auden knew that rage must be attended to, a lesson we are learning as a nation now. I never saw my father rageful, but he must have had anger at times. He tried to channel his anger into action. Into the cases he litigated. Into his work with criminal justice reform. He channeled it away from the people he loved.

At his memorial, a federal judge gave a eulogy in which he talked about Atticus Finch, Harper Lee's fictional lawyer from *To Kill a Mockingbird*. He referenced the final courtroom scene in the book, when Atticus exits and a man tells Atticus's daughter Scout to "stand up, young lady; a great man is passing by."

The judge looked out into the crowd and ended his remarks with a nearly identical refrain: "Stand up, everyone. A great man is passing."

Lea Carpenter is a screenwriter and the author of two novels: Eleven Days *and* Red, White, Blue.

In Vietnam, a Glimpse of a New Life

GEORGIA CLARK

A chance meeting with a girl at a
bar changed everything.

was sitting in a small, open-air bar in Sapa, Vietnam, wondering if I should go and talk to that girl. The American, with the loud laugh and long red hair. I assumed we were both waiting for the bus that would take us to the train that would take us back to Hanoi. Around me, tiered rice paddies cascaded down the mountainous landscape, green and lush and dramatic. Sapa is in the magnificent Northwestern region of Vietnam, a country I'd been in for about ten days. Alone. The night before I was flying here to meet up with my friend, Bec, I got an email: "So I met this guy and we're kind of in love and I'm in Mongolia. Meet us in Mongolia!"

Bec and I had been planning our trip to Vietnam and Cambodia ever since I'd decided to quit my job as the editor of a music magazine in an effort to become a writer. I was stunned and angry but, to be honest, unsurprised. Bec was fun but chronically unreliable. (Didn't we all have those friends in our twenties?) But I didn't have time to wallow. I still was going to Vietnam—but I was going alone.

I'd never traveled solo. At first, it felt strange to make every decision, from when to eat to where to sleep, on my own. But soon, it felt liberating—even decadent. I hadn't even felt lonely: the culture shock of steamy, busy Hanoi, where one crossed the street by walking into oncoming traffic with the hope it flowed around you like a water-fall of motorbikes, had been a wonderful distraction. But here in the quiet mountains, I was starting to feel like company.

Star Black—her real name—was warm and easy to talk to. She was from Brooklyn, which to me seemed as foreign and glam-orous as the moon. Back in Hanoi, she took me to a hotel rooftop bar, fancier than any of the places I'd frequented in my hometown of Sydney. We were the only ones on the plush velvet couches that offered 360-degree views of the glittery, muggy city. I ordered a Tiger beer. She ordered a Johnny Walker Blue. I'd never heard of Johnny Walker Blue. It was the most expensive thing on their menu, and it was five American dollars. "This is fifty dollars a glass back home," she said, swirling the scotch appreciatively. She wasn't pretentious: she was a sensual-ist. She wrote her email address in my travel journal, and we parted ways. My attention turned to getting to the next town, and the next, and eventually back to Australia. Star Black and her expensive whis-key faded from my mind.

I'd never traveled solo. At first, it felt strange to make every decision, from when to eat to where to sleep, on my own. But soon, it felt liberating—even decadent.

Two years later, my roommate Risha was planning a trip to New York with a couple of girlfriends. To most Sydneysiders, including myself, New York was a faraway fairytale of skyscrapers and celebri-ties. I was in. I emailed Star Black. I'd never forgotten meeting some-one from Brooklyn and thought of her every time I drank whiskey, swirling it in my glass. She wrote me back: of course she remem-bered me and better yet, she'd be away for most of my trip: would I like to cat-sit her apartment in the lovely-sounding neighborhood of Greenpoint in Brooklyn? I would.

My flight landed at 1 a.m. on a Friday in August, 2007. Right away, I was enlivened by New York, which I described as "my future home" in a gushing postcard to my parents. "It's the best city in the whole world!" I scrawled, practically panting, "I know why Sydney was becoming such a bore: I'm supposed to live here!" I saw five-dollar improv shows at UCB Theatre, gawked at MOMA's permanent collection, got lost in Central Park, and ate pizza as a snack. Greenpoint was quiet and neighborly, full of Polish restaurants and hip bars with wooden floors and kids my age with visible underarm hair. Every night, I came home to a plant-and-cat-filled apartment and started Googling "visa for America." I prayed to Buddha and God and my angels and the universe to bring me back there, please.

"This is fifty dollars a glass back home," she said, swirling the scotch appreciatively. She wasn't pretentious: she was a sensualist.

After we returned home, Risha and I moped, depressed. New York was on the other side of the planet and we were . . . not. But I stuck to my guns. I started telling everyone I was moving to New York, and to my surprise, everyone believed me. I won a national idea pitching competition, the prize of which included a return trip anywhere in the world. You can guess where I chose.

I arrived back in Brooklyn in March of 2009 with two enormous suitcases I couldn't quite carry on my own. I didn't have a visa, or a job, or a place to stay beyond a ten-day sublet. The first six months were a blur of new friends and two nudist roommates—true story—and getting hopelessly lost despite the city being a grid. But by the end of the year, I'd secured a small but cute room with two new friends in a three-bedroom apartment back in Greenpoint. As the city emptied out for Christmas, I finally got around to emailing Star Black. I couldn't remember her physical address in Greenpoint—I couldn't find it in my inbox and had no idea where my current apartment was in relation to hers. "I'm at 684 Leonard Street," I told her. "Where are you?" She emailed me right back. "Hon, I'm at 682 Leonard Street."

All those hot August nights spent praying to Buddha and God and my angels and the universe worked so staggeringly precisely, I ended up literally back in the place I fell in love with. At my local bottle shop, I bought the most expensive bottle of whiskey I could afford. Star Black and I drank it on her roof, freezing but thrilled to see each other, swirling it in our glasses as the lights of the city came on.

🕐

Georgia Clark is an author, performer, and screenwriter. She wrote the critically acclaimed novels The Bucket List *and* The Regulars, *and others. Georgia is the host and founder of the popular storytelling series* Generation Women.

This Little Sprout of Mine

DONNA HEMANS

I hoped naming my plant would help it survive.

"You killed it," my niece said.

She was looking at the terrarium in the center of my dining table. It was a glass jar made up of brownish moss, a rock, and a miniature female figurine simultaneously standing on her head and reading.

"There's still some green," I said hopefully, sprinkling a bit of water on the small tufts that clung to the glass and the rock.

I had been trying to revive it for nearly a year, avoiding the inevitable step of replacing it with a fresh evergreen carpet. Doing so would be admitting my biggest failure: I come from a family of farmers, yet most everything I plant—or any plant in my care—dies. So the terrarium suffered the same fate as the lucky bamboo plant it replaced.

This spring, especially with many of my outdoor activities off limits because of statewide lockdowns, tending a small garden was supposed to have been a mood-boosting activity. Indeed, a recent study published in the journal *Landscape and Urban Planning* says exactly that. According to the study, gardening—whether growing vegetables or ornamental plants—is as effective at boosting a person's mood as biking, walking, eating out, and other popular leisure activities. And news article after news article describe the growing interest across the country during the lockdown in growing vegetables, herbs, and fruit.

Yet, gardening has never been a mood-boosting activity for me, but rather one driven by angst and filled with worry that all my efforts will fail.

When I was a child in Jamaica, my father maintained a greenhouse in the backyard with a wide variety of anthuriums and other plants whose names I don't recall. He circumposed the croton, lychee, and citrus plants that grew in our yard, making cuttings for others who asked or replanting them around the yard. He grew callaloo, peas, peppers, yam, sweet potato, cabbage—all manner of produce that filled plates and supplemented the produce that my mother bought in the market. My father's father had done the same; farming was his livelihood. The hillside that sloped away from my grandparents' house was filled with cocoa, coffee, banana, plantain, and more.

> Gardening has never been a mood-boosting activity for me, but rather one driven by angst and filled with worry that all my efforts will fail.

Yet, here in the Washington, DC, suburbs where I live, I had failed at maintaining a simple miniature moss garden. One summer, before resorting to the terrarium, I tried container gardening, putting a tomato plant in one pot and thyme in a second. I also planted raspberry and blueberry shrubs in the middle of my townhome's small yard. That year, I reaped a handful of cherry tomatoes and raspberries before the birds took the rest. Both the raspberry and blueberry shrubs withered in the heat.

Year after year, I have attempted to replace the grass in the backyard with some kind of groundcover that requires little watering and no fertilizer. Even the clover seeds refused to grow.

Disappointed, I sat with a landscape artist to draw up a plan to replace the grass with stone and create an extension of the patio.

"What color flowers do you want?" he asked.

"Oh, I don't care about color," I said. "I just want plants that need little care."

He looked at me, successfully hiding his surprise, and carried on, changing the plants he suggested to something hardy.

I didn't use the landscaper's design. What I took from our meeting was that I needed plants that can survive on their own, plants that thrive in desertlike conditions. In the backyard, I planted hardy succulents that need little water. Some have done well, reviving each spring and defying the hot Washington summers.

For the house, I turned to a moss terrarium, which I bought on a weekend trip to Brooklyn from a now-closed shop that created miniature worlds. I pored over the scenes of life drawn from ordinary moments—a couple hiking, a woman on a park bench, a beach scene—searching for one that reflected my life. I knew, somehow, that I could maintain moss. I read the instructions, spritzed the moss every few weeks, and sometimes moved the terrarium from the dining table to the shaft of afternoon sunlight that spread across the living room floor.

Perhaps I watered it too much. Perhaps it needed less time in the sun. But it is gone now, and I am replacing the dying moss with a fresh carpet. I'm borrowing something from the Washington, DC, area and naming it after myself.

If nothing else, I have to keep my namesake alive.

Instead of gardening during lockdown, I painted small furniture and decorative pieces around my house in an attempt to bring color inside. With everything at a standstill, I wanted colors that reflected movement and growth. I painted a red wooden folding chair and a three-foot candleholder lime green, and started other projects involving coral paint and another color described as cake batter. There have been some pleasant surprises, however: a single perennial from last year's gardening attempt has bloomed again. Small fuchsia colored-flowers brighten the bed. They give me a sliver of hope, reminding me what spring should be: a celebration of rebirth and growth and the circular nature of life.

Donna Hemans is the author of the award-winning novel River Woman *and the novel* Tea by the Sea.

In Japan, a Mother and Son Find New Balance

JANICE KAPLAN

Among quiet rock gardens and bustling city intersections, I saw my son come into his own.

I thought I had passed the age when I would drop everything because a man called. And then came the moment that proved me wrong. He was traveling in Asia and he had an unexpected free week. Could I possibly join him?

The obvious answer was no. I had just started a new job with a packed schedule and many commitments.

Instead, I gave a very clear "yes."

He wanted someplace exotic, but taking many connecting flights meant I'd have only a few days, so he proposed Tokyo. He had recently been but didn't mind visiting again, and the direct flight would be easy.

I booked a ticket at the last minute and could only get a middle seat in the center section. But it didn't matter. I put on headphones when I got on the plane and closed my eyes, overcome by a wash of joy. A whole week together! However I tried to keep my heart beating calmly in my chest, it soared and floated and spiraled out among the wispy clouds. The thirteen-hour flight passed in a flash.

His flight from Hong Kong was scheduled to arrive about an hour after mine from New York, and he suggested I wait for him at a coffee shop he remembered in Terminal 2 of the Tokyo airport. I landed in Terminal 1, and by the time I found my way, I wearily wondered if this rendezvous would happen.

Then gazing across the terminal, I saw him: tall, striking, and striding quickly toward me. I had almost forgotten just how handsome he was, with a newly earned self-confidence and strength evident in every step.

I stood up, heart beating. "You found me!"

"Hi, Mom," he said.

My son, my grown-up son.

He gave me a hug and reached for my suitcase. "I'm glad you're here. I thought we'd take a train to the hotel," he said.

"You lead. I'm happy to follow."

He looked surprised. We always claim we hope our children will grow up to be strong and independent—and at some point, we have to prove we mean it. This seemed the week to let the parent-child balance change. Zach was six-foot-one, smart, and had just graduated from Yale. He was spending the summer traveling and had visited Tokyo before, which I had not. On what basis could I consider myself the natural leader of the team anymore? You never stop being a parent, but the trick is to know when your child has stopped being a child.

You never stop being a parent, but the trick is to know when your child has stopped being a child.

Zach got us onto a subway, navigating the Japanese signs, and we emerged into a vibrant neighborhood with tall buildings and throngs of people. After some freshening up, we went out to explore and then headed to a tiny sushi restaurant for dinner. Sitting at the shiny counter, we watched the chefs wielding sharp knives and then plopping their creations in front of us without plates or chopsticks.

Everyone else in the restaurant seemed to be locals and we quickly learned to dip our fingers into the pebble-strewn stream running under the counter. Two men at the very end kept watching us, and when we finished and got up to leave, they came over and shook Zach's hand. One tried out his very limited English.

"Girlfriend," he said, smiling at Zach and pointing to me.

"Mother! Mother!" I said vehemently.

The man smiled again.

"Pretty girlfriend," he said.

"Mother!" I repeated.

We left quickly, and when I told Zach how mortified I was, he just laughed. "I'm an adult, Mom," he said. "I just thought it was funny."

Over the next few days, we explored Tokyo, delighting in the bustling intersections, the endless shopping, and the many neighborhoods. Even coming from New York City, we were overwhelmed by the neon lights and the feeling of a city on steroids. But we also found a quiet shop with exquisite hand-painted kites. We ate, we talked, and we wandered. Most of all, we connected as equals.

Heading to Kyoto one day, we boarded the wrong train at the busy Tokyo station. We had just settled into our seats when Zach figured out the mistake and whisked us off just as the doors were closing. He got us to the correct train in time and looked thoroughly pleased.

Kyoto was magical, and we spent the next few days wandering through shrines and temples, taking off our shoes to slip along polished wooden floors. We learned that in Shinto shrines, you can clap your hands or ring a bell to call the gods, while Buddhism is a quieter religion. We strolled on forest trails and alongside a canal, and one afternoon in a beautifully peaceful garden, Zach looked around and clapped his hands.

We always claim we hope our children will grow up to be strong and independent—and at some point, we have to prove we mean it.

"In places like this you feel that you really could summon the gods," he said.

In that quiet setting, we talked about luck and opportunity, about setting the course for your future but still recognizing serendipity. I listened far more than I spoke, marveling at my son's insights. How had he become so wise? When he was a baby, rolling over for the first time or sitting up, I would think, *How can you do that today when you couldn't do it yesterday?* Then he got a little bigger and might use a new phrase and I would wonder, *How do you know something that I didn't teach you?* The questions never disappear; they just become more potent over time.

The next day, in another part of Kyoto, we took our buzzing American selves into a Zen rock garden. It sounded rather silly to me, but it didn't take long to be won over by the absolute peacefulness. Most gardens worship nature, but this spot had no natural beauty—just fifteen stones arranged to inspire contemplation. From wherever you stood, you could see only fourteen of them at a time. Maybe the symbolism was too obvious: However much you want to see everything, you only ever get only a partial perspective on the world. It is true of your children, too. They are your heart and soul, but the real joy is recognizing the fifteenth stone, the part not always on view.

🕐

Janice Kaplan is the former editor-in-chief of Parade *and the author of many bestselling books, including* The Gratitude Diaries: How a Year Looking on the Bright Side Can Transform Your Life. *Her latest book is* The Genius of Women: From Overlooked to Changing the World. *She hosts the podcast* The Gratitude Diaries.

Lessons from My Origami Failures

NICOLE C. KEAR

I am not crafty.

At least, not in the "whiz with a glue gun" sense. In the "cunning and wily" sense, yes, sure, I'd qualify. But all the cunning in the world won't help when you're faced with a pile of pompoms and no earthly idea how to turn them into a giraffe.

I feel the same way about crafting that I do about yoga and eliminating refined sugar from my diet. Yes, yes, a thousand times yes. Sign me up, so long as it's a theoretical sign-up, not one I have to actually go through with. Because in practice, crafting is hard. And parenting three kids in today's world is hard enough.

But life, as we know, is nothing if not unpredictable. And so I now find myself stuck at home with my three kids for an indefinite period of time, charged with their education and enlightenment. Suddenly, I have all the time in the world to do the crafts I claimed I was too busy for, in my previous, free-to-roam-the-world life.

Enter origami.

As crafts go, origami is as good as it gets. It's got a small footprint and is mess-free. All it requires is a single sheet of paper and a brain that can follow simple directions. However, I do not have that brain. I'm certain that an MRI would confirm that. So when I asked my seven-year-old what fun projects she wanted to do while we were housebound, and she replied: "Origami!" I was filled with dread.

Still, if there was ever a time to get a handle on origami, it was now. There was—there is—so much beyond my control, but this, at least, I could exercise power over.

"Let's do this," I told her.

I agreed to try a super-easy, beginner origami project—a star. The how-to video we found promised it would take under two minutes.

I didn't have origami paper but, I figured, how important could that be? Spoiler alert: very.

It took us a full five minutes to realize that an 8.5 x 11 sheet of printer paper would not yield the same results as a square piece because of, you know, geometry. Then it took another five minutes to figure out how to make squares out of rectangles.

I handed the square-ish paper to my daughter, who attempted to imitate the motions demonstrated in the video. It did take under two minutes—for her to decide the project was too hard for her, and to pass the baton to me. This had not been our agreement. But it's kind of like when I took my son to the science museum and we waited for twenty minutes so he could lie on the bed of nails and then, when it was his turn, he said he didn't want to, but he insisted I do it instead. And, naturally, I did.

Because in practice, crafting is hard. And parenting three kids in today's world is hard enough.

"Oh, honey, you do it," I told my daughter.

I am not a visual learner. The prospect of assembling an Ikea bookshelf makes my blood run cold. Puzzles make me panic. Truly. The thought that someone would take a perfectly good picture and smash it into a thousand pieces, then sell that mess to someone with the instructions, "Put this back together" thinking it could be construed as fun—that stupefies me.

"I'm terrible at origami," I said. My daughter gasped.

"Mom, you're supposed to have a growth mindset!"

(This, of course, is the trouble with educating kids. It comes back to haunt you.)

"How will you ever get good at it unless you try?" she asked, parroting words I've spoken to her.

So I tried. I mimicked the disembodied fingers on the video. They were so fast, so deft, so sure.

"How is she—" I sputtered. "I mean, do we fold up, or down? Oh my—she's going too fast! I can't do this!"

It is my understanding that origami is relaxing, meditative. This was not the case for me.

It didn't help to have my daughter providing a running commentary over my shoulder: "No, that's not right—Mom! It doesn't look anything like—Mom, Momomomom. THAT'S THE WORST STAR I EVER SAW!"

"Just—would you just hold on . . ." I paused the video, then unpaused it, then paused it again, trying to make my paper look like the one on the screen. "I think we're almost there, just one more foooooold."

It's one of the most important functions of family and friends, to help you keep moving forward, one small step at a time, to cheer you on, to tell you, "You can do it!"

But that fold, when completed, resulted in a shapeless paper blob.

"Mom," my daughter said, narrowing her eyes at me. "Mom! That's *terrible!*"

I closed my laptop and stood up.

"Let's go to bed. We can try again another time."

My daughter's face scrunched up and her eyes filled with tears. "You said our family motto is: We never give up!"

"Yes but—."

"No buts!" She must've sensed that she was gaining leverage, because she continued. "We never give up."

It is our family motto. For better or worse.

So I opened the laptop and made a fresh sheet of origami-ish paper. I watched the super speed video again. And this time, I noticed something I hadn't before.

"I know what we're doing wrong!" I shrieked, with mounting excitement. "Here—when we make this fold—see? The paper has been *upside down!*"

"*It was upside down!*" my daughter bellowed gleefully.

And then, in under two minutes, we were admiring our beautiful, though definitely not perfect, origami star.

"We did it," I said with a satisfied sigh.

"Yep," my daughter agreed.

"Aren't you glad I didn't let you give up?" I looked at her small, impertinent face.

"Yes, I am," I told her.

It was true.

It's one of the most important functions of family and friends, to help you keep moving forward, one small step at a time, to cheer you on, to tell you, "You can do it!" (or in the case of ruthless taskmaster children, to tell you, "You must do it!") when you are sure you can't.

This is always important but right now, with things so haywire, it's essential. "You were right," I told my daughter. "We never give up. Even in origami."

"Good," she nodded, satisfied. "Now let's make a whole bunch more!"

🕐

Nicole C. Kear is the author of Foreverland, The Fix-it Friends *and* The Start-Up Squad *series, and a memoir for adults,* Now I See You.

Awake: 3:01 a.m.

JOHN KENNEY

See, you say / I swimmed.

You can't swim
but insist you can.
So afraid but such courage
when you leap in
pop up
eyes wide
lost for a terrible moment
reaching for me.

See, you say.
I swimmed.

You don't know who Bobby Orr is.
Or where I went to elementary school.
Or what my mother's voice sounded like.

You are four
and it dawns on me now
Awake
that I am the exact age she was
when she died.

That's a lie.
It didn't just dawn on me.
I've always known.
Since the nurse told my father
A long time ago
pulled him aside and told my father
apparently had great difficulty getting it out
when she told my father
that my mother's last words were
I can't leave my children.

So now I stare up into the dark
thinking the same thing
about you
as the hot tears
stream down my face
into my ears
Smiling
because tears in my ears
is a phrase
that would make you laugh.

⏰

John Kenney is the New York Times *bestselling author of the humorous poetry collections* Love Poems for Married People, Love Poems for People with Children, Love Poems for Anxious People, *and* Love Poems for the Office (or Wherever), *and the novels* Talk to Me *and* Truth in Advertising, *which won the Thurber Prize for American Humor.*

Why I'm Glad No One's Driving Right Now—Including Me

SALLY KOSLOW

On life in the perpetual passenger seat.

One reason I married my husband was that not only did he own a car, he possessed a homing pigeon's internal GPS. Both of these things meant that for the duration of our relationship, I would blessedly be off the hook from ever having to get behind the wheel.

Some of my most crucial life decisions have been weighted by driving dread. After college in the Midwest, I considered moving to Chicago, Washington, DC, or Los Angeles, each a reasonably affordable, desirable destination. It was only Manhattan, however—the costliest city in the land—that called my name, strictly because its mass transportation system made it the easiest American city in which a driving weenie like myself could survive. It's been ever thus.

Now that the pandemic is keeping us sheltered-in-place, I couldn't care less about the road trips I'm not taking. I fail to understand why the fear of driving doesn't merit its own handle, like gamophobia (fear of marriage) or taphephobia (fear of being buried alive).

I can't believe I'm the only person who breaks a sweat when on the other side of a slender yellow line. Seriously: an ill-equipped individual—me, for example—is operating tons of machinery that can, with one false move, maim another human being? I have obsessed about this since long before texting was a thing.

I have now spent many years in my heroic husband's passenger seat, where, being a creative type, my mind wanders. As a result, I retain only the dimmest grasp of how to navigate the megalopolis where I live. Mosholu Parkway? The Kosciuszko Bridge? The charmingly named Sunrise Highway? These locations sound vaguely familiar, thanks to the patois of traffic alerts, but do not ask me for directions, because I literally never know where I'm going. This compounds my underlying anxiety, along with the fact that New York City's streets are home to a disproportionate number of audacious drivers who consider speed limits to be mere suggestions and who turn without signaling from whatever lane they fancy.

Some of my most crucial life decisions have been weighted by driving dread.

Given my history, you might assume I don't possess a driver's license. You would be wrong. I've been licensed to drive—and possibly kill—since I went kicking and screaming to the DMV a full year after all of my friends became certified at sixteen in my home state of North Dakota. Nonetheless, rarely did I ask to borrow the family car. Maneuver out of snowbanks? Merge with traffic? Maintain the speed limit? Not happening.

In my twenties I once found sufficient courage to drive all the way to Cape Cod, in a biblical downpour. I felt as proud as if I'd run a marathon. But unfortunately, just as I was on the cusp of becoming comfortable with driving, I caused two collisions. There was another car on the road? Really? These mishaps thoroughly obliterated my confidence and parked me, literally, on the curb for a good long while.

Recently, rational-me has tried to convince paranoid-me that not driving is barking mad, since it dramatically handicaps my independence. I can live without zipping to a suburban Costco or making a quick hop to the Hamptons on a cloudless, ninety-degree day. But I've recognized that, should I want to ditch NYC for a little respite from our urban quarantine, I'm screwed, since driving is required in any other place where I can imagine living. Thus, I have sworn to get down and dirty behind the wheel. If 227.5 million adults and teenagers in the United States can drive a car, why can't I?

My first recent foray, on a nearly deserted parkway one sunny Sunday afternoon pre-pandemic, was borderline pleasant. With my husband at my side, my terror alarm sounded only when I spotted a hell-for-leather Hells Angels brigade speeding—hand to God—directly toward my bumper.

"Right! Go! Move!" my husband shrieked as I white-knuckled the steering wheel, and then stalled the car at a busy intersection.

I was that driver, the one you curse.

Since then, with considerable practice, I've improved. Give me a country road and no need to pass a double-wide or tractor puttering along at ten miles per hour, and I will get from A to B. You would not want me to ferry your baby home from the hospital and no one will mistake me for either Thelma or Louise. But I will get the job done, even if afterward I require a day to decompress.

In times like these, that feels like enough.

Sally Koslow is the author of multiple books including Another Side of Paradise, The Widow Waltz, *and the nonfiction work* Slouching toward Adulthood. *Her debut novel,* Little Pink Slips, *was inspired by her long career as the editor-in-chief of* McCall's *magazine.*

Growing Up, Every Day Was Father's Day

MAYA SHANBHAG LANG

**In my dysfunctional Indian family,
Dad's needs always came first.**

When I was a child, we never celebrated Father's Day.

My family was Indian. We dismissed Father's Day as a strange American custom. Yet we celebrated Mother's Day each year without fail—a discrepancy that only dawns on me now that I'm in my forties.

My father, a difficult man with a temper, probably would have loved to be honored on that paternal holiday. In hindsight, it surprises me he didn't insist on it—except I think he knew my mother called the shots in our household. He could get her to go along with him in certain ways, could get her to play a part at social functions or in front of others. But had he asked her to buy a Father's Day cake, she would have laughed at him.

On Mother's Day, my father went along with whatever plans my brother and I concocted. He was strangely passive as he drove us to the supermarket. We all needed my mother. This was never to be discussed aloud, but one day a year it could be acknowledged in the form of a sticky American breakfast served in bed and a modest potted African violet placed on the tray. I doubt my mom liked what we served her, but she made a big show of her delight.

When I think about what Father's Day is supposed to be—a day when the whole family caters to the father's needs—it occurs to me that every day was Father's Day in my childhood home. He dictated what we should do. He insisted on certain forms of respect: being served first at dinner, lazing in front of the television all evening. My mom, a physician, worked longer hours than he did. She would then come home and make dinner and do the laundry and handle me and my brother while my dad relaxed. His daily life held a certain languid ease, barking out whenever he wanted a glass of water or a snack. He was served every day of his life, and he got what he wanted.

I know my dysfunctional Indian family was hardly typical. But I also wonder if our dynamic wasn't so unusual: more of a to-do on Mother's Day, little to nothing on Father's Day. This atoned for a larger pattern: My mother did too much, my father not enough.

In my own marriage, before I separated, I was showered with gifts every Mother's Day. It made me uncomfortable, though I could never say why. The gestures were thoughtful and lovely. I readied myself to exclaim in delight over the flowers and wrapped presents, reprimanded myself that other women would envy me. But deep down, some part of me dreaded the gifts. I knew they were compensatory.

> When I think about what Father's Day is supposed to be—a day when the whole family caters to the father's needs—it occurs to me that every day was Father's Day in my childhood home.

My ex-husband was nothing like my father, was never controlling or abusive, but his gifts always felt addressed to what the two of us spent all year skirting. One day was supposed to make up for all we left unsaid.

For my part, on Father's Day I showered my ex-husband with gifts right back. I threw him parties and bought him lavish presents.

I wanted to view him a certain way. Celebrating him enabled me to heighten those qualities, to think about the partner I wanted instead of the one that I had. I, too, was trying to compensate.

Now that we are separated, my ex-husband and I are solid co-parents. We may have wanted to be fifty-fifty parents while married, but it felt impossible when we lived under the same roof.

People think of divorce as a terrible outcome, but I have seen my daughter form a closer bond with her father since he and I separated. Their time together now is their own. I am not there in the background. When she is with him, she is with him. This benefits all of us. I am a far better mother because I get actual breaks. My daughter knows what it is like to have her dad's undivided attention for long stretches.

> People think of divorce as a terrible outcome, but I have seen my daughter form a closer bond with her father since he and I separated.

Maybe this Father's Day I will give my ex-husband a card. Maybe it will say something like this: We have had our differences and struggles, but I see you being a wonderful dad. You are more plugged in and engaged than ever. I am so glad.

What an awkward card that would be, not at all an array of perfectly wrapped, lovely gifts. But I find that as I get older, I would rather have awkward and true than perfect and fake.

🕐

Maya Shanbhag Lang is the author of What We Carry: A Memoir *and* The Sixteenth of June: A Novel.

Moms Don't Have Time
for the Movies

EVANGELINE LILLY

I watched the Oscars for the first time this year. Of the main half-dozen or so films being recognized, I had seen one. One! And that one I had watched under unusual circumstances.

I live in a very rural area of Hawaii. Three months ago, I drove forty-five minutes into "town" to get my hair bleached for an upcoming role. My amazing husband had the kids so they were good for as long as I needed. I knew the process would take hours and that I would be driving home during rush-hour traffic, which would double my driving time to an hour-and-a-half. So, instead of enduring the traffic, I opted to do something that felt indulgent for a working mother of two under ten: I decided to treat myself to a movie in order to wait out the traffic. There was a 6:00 p.m. showing of *Little Women* at the local four-room theater and I couldn't imagine a more perfect film to see by myself—sans husband, sans kiddies.

Time and space seemed to open up before me as I walked toward the theater and purchased my ticket from the cranky old lady who owns the joint. There were zero demands. There was nothing pressing I needed to take care of. There was even . . . wait for it . . . no sense of guilt. (Shock-face emoji.) The circumstances were such that watching this film was the only reasonable thing to do with the next couple of hours of my life, and I could feel the creep of decadent pleasure seeping into my bloodstream.

I bought a hot dog and popcorn. I ate them at my leisure without any groping little paws or begging little mouths. I saw a poster for the film *Cats* and pulled up the trailer on my phone. I was swept away in Jennifer Hudson's rendition of "Memory" without interruption, distraction, or low-lying shame for ignoring my boys. And then I watched a film so beautiful, so relevant, so poignant and life-affirming that every pore in my rapidly aging face seemed to breathe a tender sigh of yes.

I contribute to this modern world of storytelling. As a writer, I tell stories I want my children to hear. As an actress, can I say as much?

A few weeks later, I was back in the normal grind of working and mothering and wife-ing and self-caring. Since we were now in Dallas shooting the film for which I had bleached my hair, and the weather outside was more often bleak than not, my boys (including my husband) were spending a lot of time watching one of the three big screen TVs in our Airbnb.

Back in Hawaii, our kids live primarily outdoor lives. Screen time is rare, and that's how I like it. As an actress, I have to watch some content, but as a mother I find our global addiction to screens disconcerting. While I wasn't thrilled at the amount of media consumption that was happening in our temporary home, I was, at first, happy to see that our boys were watching old classics from mine and Norm's younger years: *Big*, *Three Musketeers*, and *Police Academy* were in the rotation.

If they're going to fry their brains, I thought, at least those films will have slower pacing, less graphic violence, and be more innocent than most of the "crap" they make for kids today.

Sometimes I'd get lured down memory lane and sit for a few minutes to watch with them on my way out the door to work. When I did, my stomach would drop as I realized for the first time as an adult just how acutely most of the films I adored had misshapen my little 1980s girl mind. I could not believe the overt degradation of women that I was seeing on the screens before me. Women in tight clothing with perfect hair were casually leered at, poked, groped, cat-called, and downright molested, nine times out of ten in the name of humor. I could not fathom that it was ever okay for little girls, little boys, men, and women to sit back and chuckle at men being utter pigs with no more recourse than a put-off guffaw from the women they were diminishing.

The thought crossed my mind—we have come so far.

I have a tendency to idealize my youth. The eighties with its blue-collar morality had a lot of great things to look back on and miss. But. Sitting there with my boys, I wanted to undo what was inevitably going into their brains through those actors, through that screen. I didn't want them to be able to fathom a world where disrespecting women was okay, let alone funny. I didn't want the idea of such behavior even introduced to their susceptible little psyches.

As an actress, I have to watch some content, but as a mother I find our global addiction to screens disconcerting.

Though I loathe the prevalence of screens in our modern times, I try not to censor what my kids watch too much. That may seem like a contradiction, but I believe there's a danger—a loss of oppor-tunity for independence, individuality, exposure, and identity forma-tion—when we control our children's life experiences to the letter. But as I sat there wanting to protect their minds from this toxicity, it occurred to me that I don't contribute to their film-watching experi-ences nearly enough. Frankly, I wouldn't even know where to begin. And I'm in the business.

There is so much content out there today—for us, for them—I have all but opted out. I was never much of a film and television consumer even before the content explosion of the early 2010s, but since? You can forget it. I manage one or two seasons of one or two shows a year. I probably squeak in half a dozen to a dozen films a year. As it is, I am so stretched with life and all of its constant demands that watching content takes a back seat; I treat it as something utterly unimportant.

Watching the Oscars this year, the previous few weeks really congealed inside of me. I was struck by how magical that night alone in the theater watching *Little Women* really was for me. Greta Gerwig had swept me away and left me feeling connected to the energy of every living thing—to womanhood and sisterhood, to destiny, delight, and devastation. Walking out of the theater and for the next twenty-four hours, every cell in my body was trembling with the thrill of being alive. I was struck by how acutely I had received the messages from my seemingly harmless childhood films filled with bare-chested, scantily clad women on the arms of arrogant, selfish, and cheeky men. They had stained me. They had told me what was acceptable, what was to be tolerated and what was funny. They were wrong. And I was struck by my duty to my sons: to do better by them than society had done by me. I connected to the awesome power I have as a mother to introduce art to my kids that would make them feel how I felt that night walking out of *Little Women*. I could not only usher them into a higher level of pleasure, but also help protect them from being blindly misshapen.

I contribute to this modern world of story-telling. As a writer, I tell stories I want my children to hear. As an actress, can I say as much? Truth be told, I don't think of my children when I choose the films I will participate in. I make decisions based mainly on the stories that I respond to somewhere deep inside. The little girl in me chose *The Hobbit* because thirteen-year-old Evangeline spent many a night fantasizing about being a woodland elf after reading Tolkien. I chose Marvel because it seemed like it would be a lot of fun and, Lord knows, adult Evangeline was in professional need of as much of that as possible. But did I think about the violence inherent in the characters I played and how that was contributing to the tolerance children might inherit toward violence? Not much. Not until after the films were released and part of me was dying to show my kiddies what Mommy had been a part of and another part of me didn't want my kids to see Mommy acting out violently.

I am a big contrarian, and I gave birth to a little one. My eight-year-old son knows his mommy hates violence and has been telling me since he was three years old, "Mommy, I love violence." Though it mystifies me, I have been able to recognize, over five years of allowing him to show me what he likes in content, that something in him truly responds to violence, the same way I responded to *Little Women*. It touches something visceral, deep inside of him. He's a little boy growing up in a culture where there are so few outlets for his growing testosterone and aggression. Most men don't hunt anymore. Most men don't fistfight anymore. Most men aren't even allowed to raise their voices or punch a wall anymore. But I do think aggression is in many of them. I try to watch and know his interests, even if I can't understand them, and I hope and pray that he will afford me and other women the same grace as he ages. I try to know him better through what he likes to watch, and I try to accept that the things that touch him can and will be different than the things that touch me.

I don't normally have a lot of extra time to spare, but I want to watch more films that inspire me, for my own sake, for my own soul. Not just whatever new, top ten, children's fluff Netflix is ramming down my pupils, but films that I seek out as nourishment for my depleted soul. I don't get as much time with my kids as I'd like to have, but I'd like to use some of it to learn what they respond to in movies and use that information to find worthwhile, beautiful content that we can watch together to stimulate conversations about our interests and values, to better understand one another. And now, while we're all at home from work and school together, is a perfect time to practice.

I am taking turns with my sons.

"Let's watch a movie I like and then you can choose a movie you wanna see. Let's watch both together and let's talk about them after."

It sounds so simple, it sounds so small, but it can be powerfully bonding and formative, and it accomplishes that ever-so-important mommy virtue: checking multiple things off the mommy-priority list in one fell swoop.

Self-care: Check.

Child-bonding: Check.

Child-teaching: Check.

Rest: Check.

Joy: Check.

Learning: Check.

Growth: Check.

Admittedly, I don't always love what screens have brought into our lives, but I do accept that my sons love them and that they will always be a part of our lives. So rather than opt out, I want to contribute to the habits and tastes they form in relationship to these ever-present devices. Story-telling has always been how we shape our young and how we remind ourselves. I want to remember, I want to tell my kids the right stories and I want to be there to watch their faces light up with the life that truly good stories contain.

Screens don't have to be all bad. A lonely fire in the jungle can attract predators to a solitary child sitting, unsuspecting, beside it. I don't want screens to be my babysitters. But a communal fire that we sit around together, with song and dance, stories and dramas, masks and costumes, food and drink, well . . . that fire not only scares away the predators, but it builds the family and the community. If movies, our modern-day fires, help inspire that kind of nurturing and that kind of connection, then by all means. It's time for me to make time for movies.

⊕

Evangeline Lilly is an actress best known for her roles in the TV show Lost *and the* Ant-Man *movie series. She is the author of* The Squickerwonkers *children's book series.*

Kyle and Zibby: Stepfather, Step Right Up

ZIBBY OWENS

On listening, learning, and rolling with the punches.

When Kyle and I first got together almost five years ago, all I could do was hope that my four kids would see how special he was and take to him like I had. I also hoped that he would be able to put up with them. I got lucky; I couldn't believe how effortlessly Kyle adapted to the role of stepdad. Going from zero to four kids must have been quite an emotional adjustment, but for him, he always said he was "living the dream." We sat down for our quarantine Instagram Live show *KZ Time* last month to talk about stepparenting and more.

The following are excerpts from our conversation edited for length and clarity.

Zibby Owens: Kyle is our guest today, because Father's Day is around the corner and we have to start thinking about gifts. What do you want for Father's Day?

Kyle Owens: Just to hang out with you and the kids. That's what it's all about—it's the little things nowadays. Maybe a trip to Starbucks for social distancing coffees.

Zibby: That's easy. *(To audience)* So for those for those of you who don't know, I have four kids with my previous husband.

Kyle: And I have eight kids with my previous wife.

Zibby: No, stop it! Kyle has not been married before and graciously entered into this situation and took me with all the kids in tow, which was a big ask. Before the pandemic, we had sort of a system going. The kids would go to my ex-husband's every other weekend for a long weekend. Kyle and I were able to travel. He has a career in LA as a producer, and so we spent time out there. We could take trips and go to brunch and do things as if we were young and fun. He is somewhat young, but I am feeling not so young. Now here we are in the pandemic, and we have been at home with the kids nonstop.

Kyle: Nonstop, no help.

Zibby: I should also say Kyle has been doing all the cooking. I make breakfast and smoothies and French toast and things like that.

Kyle: You work a blender well.

Zibby: Thank you. Kyle does all the dinners and most of the lunches. *(To Kyle)* You were in your early thirties when you met me. You had not had kids before. You had not been married. Then all of a sudden, you married me and inherited these four kids as a stepdad, something that maybe you hadn't considered being, or maybe you had. I don't know.

> The role of a stepparent is to roll with the punches in a lot of ways. You don't get a lot of credit for the good things that you do.

Kyle: I mean, I knew about the kids before we got married.

Zibby: My question is, in all seriousness, how did you decide that that would be okay to do? How did you come to terms with the fact that in order to be with me you would have to also live with the four kids most of the time? Then how did you figure out how to deal with it?

Kyle: I've been teaching tennis for a really long time, a lifetime if you will, and teaching little kids, kids of all ages, so I was really comfortable around kids and really comfortable communicating with kids.

Zibby: But it's different having a kid on a tennis court for half an hour and working on their forehand.

Kyle: Yeah, it was a big learning curve of just trying to find my place and my role. It obviously is much different than teaching tennis lessons. I know at the time you had been a parent already for eight years. I was trying to catch up and trying to not only go on my own instincts, learn from you, but I think most importantly, learn from the kids. Listening to them is the biggest thing for me. Today, our littlest guy was yelling at me. He wanted the soap to wash his hands. I said to him, "Look, I know you're the youngest and a lot of times you have to yell for everyone else to acknowledge that you're just talking." I said, "I'm always listening to you, so you don't have to yell at me. You can just talk to me normally in a normal voice. I'll listen to you. I'll always listen to you." He said, "Thank you. That was really nice. But I still need the soap."

My parents are both divorced and remarried . . . I almost didn't want to get close to my stepparents for a while because I felt disloyal about it.

Zibby: I have to confess that I can be very controlling with the kids, well, probably in general. I like to be in charge. I like to do things my way. I always change plans. I have a lot of weaknesses as a person and as a parent. Kyle is very laid back, which is a blessing because otherwise it doesn't work so well. If you were as aggro as I am, it would probably create a lot of conflict. I feel like you have made me a better parent, though, because you slow down when I am revved up all the time. You're always saying that you're just trying to make these kids into better people and one thing at a time. You try to appreciate the fun and do things a little differently and let things unfold organically. I was not of that mentality before. Yet I've adopted it.

Kyle: Have you?

Zibby: I mean, more so. But back to stepparenting, though.

Kyle: The role of a stepparent is to roll with the punches in a lot of ways. You don't get a lot of credit for the good things that you do. You get a lot of the blame for the bad things that you do. You're like the quarterback. If you win, everyone's like, you're great. If you lose, you're a bum. But I have learned that these kids—your kids, everyone's kids—they're just still developing their brains. They're not really as emotionally there as they will be eventually.

Zibby: Very true. And now we've been married three years. Things moved very quickly at the beginning. From the first minute, I said, "I'm not having any more kids, so you should probably just walk away right now and go and marry some pretty young thing and have your own family." *(To audience)* I never would've seen this coming. Kyle was this young, dashing, tennis pro partying in Montauk. I was bogged down with four kids and crying in the shower and all the rest of it.

Kyle: I was swinging from the rafters of the Surf Lodge.

Zibby: Somehow it all worked out.

Kyle: Getting back to the stepdad thing, which was a little easier for me because the two little ones were so little that they don't even remember, really. They don't remember anything about that time. They don't remember meeting me. To be fair, they don't really remember you being married to their dad.

Zibby: They have actually asked me if I know him sometimes. "Do you know my dad?"

Kyle: That's funny. "Have you ever met my dad before?"

Zibby: I have. I have met your dad.

Kyle: It's really cute. I think they were really into me because I was just listening to them and hanging out with them. I think that they took to it pretty well. I think because the kids pick up on your happiness, Zibby, and recognized you being happy. I think that all they want is for you to be happy regardless of if it was with me or whomever. I think they have respect for the person who's there helping that happiness grow.

Zibby: All I think about is how to protect them, especially now, and to make sure they're okay and happy. It can be hard. I sometimes lose my temper, but it's not okay for you to lose your temper because they don't respond to it the same way. There are different rules for both of us, which I think creates a lot of conflict.

Kyle: The mom and the dad, whatever they do, they're the mom and the dad. I feel like the stepmom or the stepdad, we are constantly earning respect. They're always going to listen to you when it comes down to it. They're always going to listen to their dad.

Zibby: Sorry about that. My parents are also divorced, so I relate a lot to my kids and how they feel about everything. My parents are both divorced and remarried. They split up when I was fourteen and my brother was eleven. I had to go through all the same stuff. I almost didn't want to get close to my stepparents for a while because I felt disloyal about it.

Kyle: It's a roller coaster of emotions. It's definitely amplified now during quarantine when we're just around each other twenty-four/seven. Eventually, they'll all be out of the house and in college and having their own lives. We'll be looking back on these times and probably really pining for them.

Zibby: Or not. [laughs] I'm kidding.

Kyle: But really I'm in a good spot with these kids, in all honesty. They're really cool to me. They could be terrible. I'm sure there are probably a lot of people out there who are in similar situations that I'm in, whether it's a stepmom or a stepdad, and maybe the kids are just not having it and they're not into it. I can't even imagine what that must be like.

Zibby: I'm lucky to have a loving, understanding husband in Kyle. I know. I am so lucky. Kyle is a godsend. The fact that he is so patient with the kids—four kids, and they all have moods!—it can be a lot. He's really patient. I don't want to give any illusion that we have this perfect situation. Everybody has challenges. I don't want to pretend that we don't squabble every so often. We're just like everybody else. So one more thing: If there was somebody out there who was about to be a stepparent, what advice would you give them?

Kyle: I would just say listen. You've got to listen to the kids. I would also say that the idea is not to replace someone else. Obviously, if that person is still living and is still in the picture and they're a nice person, there's no reason to feel like you're trying to ever replace that person. You're just trying to add to something already great.

Zibby Owens is a writer and mother of four in New York City. She is a literary advocate and the creator and host of the award-winning literary podcast Moms Don't Have Time to Read Books. *She runs a literary salon with author events, a virtual book club, and a daily* Z-IGTV *live author interview series.*

Next Steps: A Perfectionist Tackles the Unknown

MARY LAURA PHILPOTT

Last year, when I was on book tour for *I Miss You When I Blink*, there was one question I heard from audiences more than any other. The first time someone asked, I was speaking to a group of investment bank employees at a corporate book club. A young woman in the second row raised her hand: "If you could go back and give your younger self one piece of advice, what would it be?"

"Quit more things," I said. "I'd tell my younger self that she didn't have to stick out every commitment she made. If you're doing something you hate—a habit you've grown tired of or a job you can't stand—stop doing it, so you can make time to do what you love instead."

I'll never forget what happened next. I wish I'd had a camera to record the crowd's reaction. Most people just nodded politely, but a handful of faces throughout the room absolutely lit up. I wondered later if a few of those investment bankers might have gotten out of investment banking afterward, and if it might have been my fault. Oops.

As a recovering perfectionist, I still have a tendency to finish everything I start. I can't help it. I like the sight of a list with every line crossed out, the feeling of being finished. But it's one thing to spend an hour watching to the end of a movie you don't love that much. It's quite another to spend a decade working in a job that makes you feel like you're sleepwalking, to live in a place you don't feel connected to anymore, or to keep up a relationship that has long since stopped serving you well.

Those of us with type-A tendencies often have to be nudged to let go, and that's how I treated this question—as a chance to tell anyone in the room who was holding on, white-knuckled, to something they needed to release that it's okay to quit and make space for what's next in their life. One of my favorite parts of each event was the book-signing line, when at least one or two people would lean in to whisper what they wanted to quit and what they dreamed of doing next. "I'm leaving my law practice and going back to school to be a counselor," one said. "I'm opening a bakery," another confided. I may have been the first to hear about a few divorces.

Now, we find ourselves in a strange time to contemplate the idea of "what's next?" With so many plans on hold as we grapple with unprecedented life-and-death questions, who dares consider the future?

We all must.

First, of course, we must do what needs doing in this moment. Care for loved ones. Mourn our losses. Check on neighbors. Donate to support those in need. But on the back burners of our minds, it's okay to keep dreams simmering. We have to believe that.

I'm a big fan of the phrase, "If you can see it, you can be it." Six years of working in a bookstore, for example, changed my writing life; being around books and writers and readers every day for years demystified the writing and publishing process. One of these days, it'll be time to get up close to your dream, so you can see it. If, say, you've been thinking about pursuing a graduate degree, perhaps now's a good time to research some programs. When you envision next year or the next, you might picture volunteering in a field that uses that

As a recovering perfectionist, I still have a tendency to finish everything I start.

degree. How might you get near to the people who are living that life to see how it looks and feels up close? To entertain such thoughts is to give yourself a reprieve from our current reality.

I often imagine conversations among my selves at different ages. (Please tell me I'm not the only one?) When I try to imagine what my future self would say to right-now-me, I'm stumped. I'm not so sure anymore that I can imagine what the future looks like. I suspect she might say, "Keep going. Keep planning." She'd want me to be careful. She'd want me to

Now, we find ourselves in a strange time to contemplate the idea of "what's next."

take care of myself and others. But she'd want me to daydream, too. I think she'd want me to take some comfort and joy today in thinking about tomorrow.

Tomorrow's what we're living for, isn't it?

Mary Laura Philpott is the author of I Miss You When I Blink: Essays, *now available in paperback. Formerly of Parnassus Books, Mary Laura has contributed to the* New York Times *and many other publications.*

Does My Daughter Miss Her Babysitter Too Much?

JULIE SATOW

**The heartbreak of social distancing
from a beloved caregiver.**

One day about a month ago, I was doing one of my endless rounds of laundry when I walked past my daughter's desk on the way to pick up her dirty clothes. Lying next to her keyboard was a lined sheet of notebook paper with the word "Penny" prominently written in blue marker.

That's the name of our babysitter, and I bent to pick up the page thinking it was a letter my daughter might want me to send. But as I gave it a quick scan, I realized it was something else entirely. "Her hair is curly/and her face is pretty," read the first line, "But that is not all/She gives the best hugs and kisses/And makes you feel better."

My nine-year-old had written a love poem to her caregiver.

Like so many other children across the world, my daughter has been whipsawed by the changes to her life over these past several months. There's been the transition to remote learning, having both working parents at home, and the realization that her younger brother is her sole IRL companion for the foreseeable future. She has brushed off most of these alterations, save for one: the sudden breach in her daily interactions with Penny. It's the single aspect of our new reality that most devastates my daughter, a persistent sense of loss that I am unable to assuage.

Our babysitter came into our life nearly a decade ago when my daughter was just a few months old. She regularly picks up our children from school, shuttles them to lessons and appointments, and over the years, the three of them have developed their own traditions, jokes, and favorite activities.

The pandemic has revealed what constitutes family, and where those lines are drawn.

I know that I am blessed. My family is healthy and safe, my marriage is strong, and my husband and I are gainfully employed. We are also fortunate to be able to employ a babysitter to help with our childcare when so many other families cannot. While I am at work, I am secure knowing that my children are being showered with affection and care, and that they are gaining so much from this relationship. Penny is a grandmother, an immigrant from Guyana, and they learn an inestimable amount from her deep life experiences.

Penny lives with her daughter, who works as a nurse at an old-age home in Brooklyn, one that was inundated with COVID-19 patients. Since the outbreak of the pandemic, as we have done with so many of our loved ones, we have kept our distance.

My husband and I both grew up with working mothers and with a succession of babysitters. There was one who got drunk and wandered off for several hours, leaving my brothers and me to fend for ourselves, while another took it upon herself to explain sex to me, years before I was ready for such a conversation. But while there were some who made bewilderingly bad decisions and I was glad when they left, others were well-loved. One, aptly named Joy, was my favorite. I recall happily spending hours with her as she told us stories of her upbringing or took us on car ride adventures around town.

When I became pregnant, I hoped to find a babysitter who would be firmly in the latter camp, and over the years, Penny became akin to a third parent. Our trust runs deep. She is the one with whom I can leave the children and be entirely off the clock—no need to text about what to make them for dinner or where to pick them up, as she often knows better than I. Penny is my partner, my closest equivalent. Our families are also intertwined. Her daughter has cared for my grandmother; her sister and niece stayed for a summer with us, and her grandchildren and our children are of similar ages and have sleepovers.

I should not have been surprised then, weeks into our quarantine, when my daughter suddenly broke into heaving sobs because she was desperate for a hug from Penny. Or when, after one of their many FaceTimes, she got off the call with a look of anguish and told me she would rather have no contact with Penny than rely on this pitiful semblance of a virtual one. When a care package arrived with bread and cakes that Penny had baked, my daughter ate a few bites before pushing away the rest, telling me it made her too sad.

I felt grateful that my daughter had such a bond, yet also exasperated that my presence was not sufficiently comforting.

These reactions stirred a mix of emotions in me. I felt grateful that my daughter had such a bond, yet also exasperated that my presence was not sufficiently comforting. My husband suggested that Penny had become symbolic of a greater loss, a representation of the normalcy that is no longer, a reminder of how my daughter's daily life had been upended. By focusing on a single person, it was easier for my daughter to process and articulate her many complex feelings. All of this may well be true. But to chalk up my daughter's emotions to such a shorthand would diminish Penny's importance. The truth is that my daughter also simply, profoundly, misses her.

Much has been said of how this pandemic has laid bare America's numerous systemic ills, from the racial disparities of COVID-19, to the horrors of George Floyd's murder, to the millions of newly jobless. Yet it has also revealed truisms in the smallest sense, down to the minutiae of the family unit.

This age of coronavirus has not merely disrupted my family's logistical balancing act, forcing us to work and learn from home, with all the difficulties that it entails. It has also fractured our family's emotional makeup. The pandemic has revealed what constitutes family, and where those lines are drawn. If, before COVID-19, I considered Penny our beloved babysitter, I have come to understand that she is much more. While it may have been my daughter who wrote a love poem to her, I cannot help but realize that now I have, too.

🕐

Julie Satow is a journalist and the author of The Plaza: The Secret Life of America's Most Famous Hotel.

AUTHOR FEATURES

AT HOME WITH

Compiled by Carolyn Murnick

Janelle Brown

Eight years ago, I cofounded a collective workspace for writers in Los Angeles with a few of my friends. It's not just the place where I wrote my new suspense novel, *Pretty Things*, it's also been my social hub and my support system.

But for the time being, my office is just a memory. My kids are home all day, and therefore so am I, which means that any writing I'm doing has to be within the confines of our property. Luckily spring is here, which means I'm able to work in fresh air.

I spend my days moving from spot to spot around our home—wherever I can get motivated (and find a few moments of peace). Sometimes I sit at a table in our garden, right under the blooming jasmine, or lie on our outdoor couch, but the kids usually find me fast. Trust me—it's hard to get in the writing zone when you're constantly being asked for snacks.

So when I really need quiet, I go lock myself in the studio at the back of our property. We built a desk under a big barn window that I throw open for fresh air; from here, I can even get a glimpse of the Hollywood sign. This is where I'm doing all my virtual book launch events for *Pretty Things*, and if you attend one, you might even hear the birds chirping in the trees just outside that window. Until I can get my real officemates back, they aren't such a bad substitute.

✦

Janelle Brown is the New York Times *bestselling author of* Watch Me Disappear, All We Ever Wanted Was Everything, *and* This is Where We Live. *Her latest book,* Pretty Things, *is being adapted into a television series starring Nicole Kidman.*

Dan Peres

If you're reading this, consider it proof of life. My small home office has been hijacked. I have to write this quickly, before my captors come back. They just stepped out of the room for a few minutes. I hear them in the kitchen just outside of the door, laughing and plotting and eating Goldfish. I can practically make out the sound of crumbs hitting the floor.

There are three of them—all male—with overgrown hair and mischievous smiles that reveal missing teeth. I'm pretty sure the two younger ones are twins—maybe nine—and they've been torturing me by "practicing" playing their recorders for an end-of-the-school-year concert that will never happen. I've been trying to write, but writing when the hostage takers are around is a bit like eating soup while riding a bicycle down a flight of stairs. This is the most I've written in two months. No need to send help, though. Maybe it's Stockholm Syndrome, but despite the incessant noise and interruptions and around-the-clock snacking, I wouldn't trade this for anything. I could, however, do without the recorders.

✦

Dan Peres is a veteran magazine editor and the author of As Needed for Pain: A Memoir of Addiction.

Lauren Mechling

It's a monastically simple setup: computer, chair, coffee. When I think about it, though, I'm filled with delight and a little smugness for having crept out of bed before anybody else in the household. It's just me and the early morning light—no sounds, no hungry bodies, no emails coming in from points unseen, those tempting vectors of distraction.

Here is my golden hour—sometimes closer to two hours—when I can sit still and string sentences together. The thing about self-isolation with two small children whose homeschooling requires hands-on oversight is that I no longer have the isolation needed to concentrate. I'm juggling a few projects, a mix of fiction and journalism, and during the day I can take breaks to conduct interviews or answer emails. The writing, though, happens before 7 a.m. I've always been a morning writer, but never has this ritual felt so urgent, or so pleasurable. It's as if I'm getting away with something.

Lauren Mechling is a journalist and author of How Could She: A Novel.

Rochelle Weinstein

Quarantine moved my writing space from Miami, Florida to Beech Mountain, North Carolina. I went from a vibrant, densely populated city to the rural mountains where the nearest Target is fifty miles away.

The cooler temperatures provide hours of writing overlooking layered, lush mountains. Deer pass, birds squawk, and dogwoods rustle in the wind. It's exquisite. But I confess, I've gone days without showering; morning to night spent in my pajamas. I've survived on Milk Duds and Twizzlers and been startled by bees and snakes. Soon, I plan to sleep on my deck, capturing every sound and sensation for an upcoming scene I'm working on.

The quarantine has sucked—let's be real. Being told you can't do something is almost as bad as not doing it. Yet lockdown has returned many of us to simpler times. It doesn't get any simpler (or more inspiring) than creating while nestled in nature under a cozy blanket.

🕐

Rochelle Weinstein is the bestselling author of novels including Somebody's Daughter, Where We Fall, The Mourning After, *and* What We Leave Behind.

POSTCARD FROM THE PAST

Compiled by Carolyn Murnick

Megan Angelo

Before there was my summer of *Hamilton*, there was my summer of *Felicity: An American Girl*. I went to Williamsburg's official Felicity tour. I was in Virginia with my whole family, but only my mom and her trusty fanny pack came with me for this part. My two younger brothers are no doubt on a bench in the shade somewhere, furious that we are somehow still not at Busch Gardens, while my father picks a fight with "Thomas Jefferson" over perceived historical inaccuracies in his spiel.

🕐

Megan Angelo is the debut author of Followers. *Her writing has appeared in the* New York Times, *where she helped launch comedy coverage, the* Wall Street Journal, Glamour, Elle, *and many other publications.*

Alice Berman

People say that Montana is "the last, best place," and they are absolutely right. I have been heading out West every summer since I was two years old. Some of my earliest memories are here, trout fishing in a sundress and burning marshmallows on the side of a mountain. My family members have long been acolytes of the beauty of Paradise Valley, where my sister and I would conveniently forget the learnings of years of English riding lessons and execute all of the daredevil jumps no one should do. (My sister was famous among the group of families we went with for bending off her horse so far she could pick flowers.) There is no comfort like the wind in the flickering silver aspen leaves, the smell of woodsmoke after a long ride, the endless stretches of empty green land.

This year, of course, we are lucky enough to be staying home and staying safe, still monitoring the weather in our favorite place as if we're going—it snowed there the day we would have arrived. My family group chat is filled with updated COVID-19 numbers for Montana and photos of the wilderness there. There is such comfort and normalcy in sharing this, in knowing that this genuine paradise is waiting patiently for us. In the meantime, I'm rereading *A River Runs Through It*, which is worth a perusal even if you've never considered Montana of interest. To me, it will always be my best place.

⊕

Alice Berman is the author of the Audible Originals mystery I Eat Men Like Air. *She sold her book,* Lost Boys and Technicolor Girls, *to ABC, where it is in development to become a series with Freeform.*

Casey Schwartz

I was hideously jetlagged on my trip to India. I had taken an Ambien the night before and, mysteriously, it hadn't worked. I walked through Kolkata that day in a kind of dream state, in awe of its particular atmosphere, its grandeur, its decay. It was January 2016, and I was thirty-three, single, and anxious. I was traveling with my mother. By the end of that year, Trump would be elected, and I would meet my husband.

I think I had the impression that it would somehow always be possible to venture through the streets of Kolkata, to see every inch of the world. Now, all I can think about is how utterly precious it was to glimpse even that ordinary, crumbling building.

⊕

Casey Schwartz is a journalist and the author of Attention: A Love Story.

Teresa Sorkin

We were in Positano, at Il San Pietro. We had just finished dining on the most amazing lunch of local mozzarella and fresh tomatoes with basil. I can still smell the lemon trees that surround the property and feel the cool breeze from the ocean air.

Unfortunately, our beloved Italy was one of the first countries after China to be devastated by the coronavirus pandemic, with nearly thirty-five thousand deaths thus far.[1] Today, they are in a better place after enduring four months of strict quarantine and have recently opened their country to most visitors, but US travelers are currently prohibited. While it breaks my heart not to return this year, I know that we will one day be back and Italy will be better than ever, as the famous song "Come Back to Sorrento" goes.

⊕

Teresa Sorkin is a television producer and coauthor of the thriller The Woman in the Park.

---

[1] Number at time of original publication.

AFTERWORD & ACKNOWLEDGMENTS

The acknowledgments section is usually the first thing I read when I start a book. I love getting that inside peek into an author's mind: their writing process, inner circle, and general thoughts. It usually reveals a lot about their personality and infuses the story with an added layer of meaning. If you don't typically read the acknowledgments page, you should! You can start with mine. Actually, look, you already did. Fantastic!

Thank you to everyone I mention below. Here's my story.

First: Kyle. My life started over at forty when I married Mr. Kyle Owens on the tennis court of a rental home. I am grateful every day—even the days I'm in a snippy mood—that he and I get to do this whole thing together. Three years ago, as we were hanging out in what became my office and used to be our shared den (sorry, love), he said, "You know, you should really take all those parenting essays you're writing and make them into a book." I sighed, rolled my eyes, and said, "Moms don't have time to read books!" Then I laughed and said, "Wait, that's what the title should be!"

Well, turns out the people I asked didn't think publishers would find that funny. They also said "essay collections don't sell" and that I needed "more of a platform." Although I'd been freelancing since I was fourteen years old, it didn't pass muster. I wasn't even on Instagram.

At the same time, I gave a speech at my kids' school about how I used to be shy but that I'd found my voice through writing. A fellow mom and bestselling author in the audience, Sarah Mlynowski, grabbed me in the hall after and say, "We should talk. Let's get coffee." (She's now one of my closest friends.) I told her about the feedback I'd been getting about my book idea. She thought about it and later, passing each other at drop-off one morning, called out, "You should start a podcast"! I yelled back, "A what?"

I went home and sat on the couch with Kyle as we tried to figure out how to find the podcast button on our phones. I Googled "how to start a podcast," researched and listened to many, and then realized that I had the perfect title already picked out. But what should the podcast be about?

I'm someone who is constantly tearing articles out of the paper and forwarding essays to friends. I'm also always reading and recommending books. (For my bridal shower to Kyle, friends were all asked to give me books.) My first thought was to narrate my favorite essays or sections of books I'd loved for mom friends who didn't have time to even read them.

Then, at coffee with books editor Mackenzie Dawson in the *New York Post*'s dining room, I found out that that was illegal. (Thanks, Mackenzie.) I figured I could try just interviewing authors directly. I knew, like, two authors. I started with my Harvard Business School classmate and dear friend, author Lea Carpenter, who had also helped me edit the novel I wrote after we graduated, *Off Balance*, that ultimately didn't sell. Next, Kyle's old colleague and close friend, former French Open champion Murphy Jensen, put me in touch with Andre Agassi, who he had just sat next to on an airplane. And Andre said yes! With those two as my first guests, I was on a roll. Friends started putting me in touch with their author friends. Before I knew it, my podcast hit the charts.

As Lea was walking out of my apartment that first day after doing her interview, she told me that soon publicists would find me, and I'd have books piling up at my doorstep. I was like, "Yeah, right."

Um, yes. Fortunately, the pitches mostly pile up in my inbox now, but for a while I couldn't even open up the boxes fast enough. Word had spread.

But back to the beginning. At coffee with Meredith Rollins, a mutual friend who had recently published an essay of mine in *Redbook,* she mentioned that she could put me in touch with her friend Dani Shapiro, who just happened to be my favorite author of all time. I told Meredith to invite Dani as my guest to the upcoming Library Lunch I was cochairing for the New York Public Library. Dani accepted the invite! I sat her next to me and even mentioned her in my beg-for-donations speech at what NYPL President Tony Marx calls "the liiiiiibrary." She came on my podcast soon after and, as she was walking out that same front door of mine, told me about an author salon series she had gone to and suggested I start doing similar in-person events. She even volunteered to be my first guest.

I moved quickly. A few weeks later, I'd organized a book fair in my home at which I decided to sell all the books I'd featured on the podcast so far. BookHampton provided the books—and took all the profits, as I intended. I invited everyone I knew in New York plus all the authors I'd featured on the podcast for a holiday shopping and meet-'n-greet style event in my home. Dani was the featured speaker along with Piper Weiss. We've been close ever since. Dani's strength going through her husband Michael's cancer inspires me to this day.

From there, things took off. Authors put me in touch with friends. They recommended that their journalist colleagues write about me. They introduced me to editors and brought me to events. Author Piper Weiss asked me to interview her at a BookHampton bookstore event when her interviewer canceled at the last minute. I realized I loved doing live events, too. Jamie Brenner invited me to interview her at Barnes & Noble, which was an enormous thrill, followed by other authors like Nicola Harrison, Brenda Janowitz, Greer Hendricks, Rochelle

Weinstein, even Candace Bushnell. I sponsored Author's Night for the East Hampton Library. I put on events at the Center for Fiction with Deborah Copaken, Lauren Mechling, and Carolyn Murnick. Lauren, by the way, recommended me for a feature article to her friend, journalist Hillary Kelly, who ended up profiling me in *Vulture*, anointing me "New York's Most Powerful Book-fluencer." That article, which I read on my phone frozen in shock on 77th and Lex, put me on the map.

Author Laurie Gelman, who I met through the fabulous Patricia Eisemann at Henry Holt (who I got to through Pamela Paul of the *New York Times Book Review*), asked me to host a book club to showcase her new book, *You've Been Volunteered*, on ABC-7 with Sandy Kenyon, an entertainment journalist I'd been watching on TV my entire life. Sandy and his wife, Eileen, have been enormous supporters of mine. In fact, Sandy came back to cover my next book fair and even put a profile piece about me on Taxi TV.

Riding in his cab, Tony Lyons, CEO of Skyhorse Publishing, saw my piece and asked his colleague Mark Gompertz to reach out to me. The three of us had coffee at Ralph's, the Ralph Lauren store coffee shop on 72nd and Madison. I heard about their unique publishing model and how quickly they were able to get books on shelves versus the glacially slow process of other publishers. I stored that info in my back pocket.

Meanwhile, I'd hired Bobby Grossman of Media One Management to help me recommend books on TV, a reference from journalist Margaret Hoover who I met through Alyssa Litoff. Bobby connected me to Ali Ehrlich from *Good Morning America*. I went back to meet Ali and her colleague, Simone Swink. Over time I became a monthly columnist for *Good Morning America* online, recommending each month's latest crop of books. He also connected me to Vidya Singh at CBS News. I was lucky enough to have Dana Jacobson interview me for a career-turning seven-minute feature on "CBS This Morning." During the pandemic, Vidya and Dana updated the piece to showcase the many ways I was helping during lockdown and released another 7-minute piece. Bobby also secured me regular spots on shows like *Good Day DC, Good Day Dallas, Good Day LA,* and others. I was moving and shaking. I couldn't believe it! Even *O, the Oprah Magazine,* included me in a list of top literary podcasts. Twice!

I say all this to thank everyone who played a part in taking the podcast, which I started one quiet morning in my bedroom with the door closed, talking into my phone, and making it into what it has become with two million downloads and countless connections to authors—people!—I never would have met. My days are filled with intimate conversations, one-on-one, about people's lives, emotions, feelings, work, and families. It's a dream come true. Sometimes I get nervous, like when interviewing superstars like Nicholas Sparks, Mitch Albom, Natalie Portman, and Alicia Keys (!), but mostly I just get excited. This is what I do. I can talk to anyone. I love to hear what they have to say.

In my introduction to this book, I explained how this anthology came to be with the enormous help of three authors/editors: Claire Gibson (who I met at Books are Magic at an event we were both attending for John Kenney and Courtney Maum), Elissa Altman (who I met through Dani Shapiro), and Carolyn Murnick (who came on the podcast and did the Center for Fiction event with me). They edited all the pieces in this book. So did my right-hand woman Jamie Mortimer, who not only helps me take care of my kids but also helps me take care of my life. I rarely do anything without asking her opinion, including my book titles, the logistics of the day, and even my outfits. A former English major, Jamie hopped in and started copy editing when lockdown kept us apart.

Maxi Kozler, who saw me speak at a Child Mind Institute benefit, ended up becoming my COO for several months pre-pandemic (and before I downsized the entire operation to its bare bones basics again). Alice Berman, a family friend and author on my podcast, came on board to help with partnerships. Katie Mitchell, my kids' chess teacher, saw me freaking out over how much I had to do one day, and offered to help. My kids' weekend babysitter, Nina Vargas, started helping, too, and ended up becoming head of my events and then, in the pandemic, my social media maven. McCain Merren, a friend of Claire Gibson's from Nashville, started filming events for me, with Kyle helping direct and produce. McCain ended up producing all my Instagram Live videos in the pandemic and the entire *We Found Time* magazine, which Somsara Rielly, my old colleague from my Vigon/Ellis days (my first job after college) designed. Kiirsten Lederer produced my podcast from the beginning after I found her through Jenny Galluzo at the Second Shift when Beth Kojima, an old friend, connected me. I couldn't function without Kiirsten's help. My oldest and best friend, Genevieve McCormack ("Aunt Gen" to my kids) did all the legal work, including every single contract for the authors in this book. She has gotten me through life since we met at age fourteen. She will forever be my "To'F" and me, her "eke." Jackie Eckhouse helped with the rest of my contracts.

After a crazy night during UN Week last year when I literally ran across the Central Park transverse to get to my daughter's kindergarten curriculum night on time, I met a fellow class mom, Vern Li. I sent around an essay the next day about my ridiculous run through the park and she asked if I had an agent. I didn't then. She introduced me to Joe Veltre, who sat in the office next to hers at Gersh, and he enthusiastically agreed to represent me. Now we've sold four books together.

Speaking of agents, when I was first getting the podcast started, I joined Twitter. The next time I checked my account, I had five followers, one of whom was a literary agent, Rachel Horowitz. I messaged her on Twitter and thanked her for being a follower and asked how she'd even found me. Turns out we had some mutual friends and were also school moms together with kids in different grades. She signed on as my agent before Joe and helped me write a memoir . . . which became a novel . . . which became a doorstop called *40 Love*. Who knows. Maybe I'll go back to it. She left her firm to take a job at HarperCollins, but remains one of my most trusted resources.

As my events at home grew, I got to know many authors more intimately, interviewing them in front of a group of friends on my couch, sipping coffee together. Many other authors attended events as guests, too. A lot of those "salon" authors have essays in this collection, such as Jill Santopolo, Gretchen Rubin, Wendy Walker, John Kenney, Liz Astrof, Lea Carpenter, Jan Eliasberg, Lauren Mechling, Janice Kaplan, Eilene Zimmerman, Rachel Levy Lesser, and Elissa Altman.

Other authors I've done live events with include Allison Pataki, Lori Gottlieb, Abby Maslin, Brenda Janowitz, Courtney Maum, Rochelle Weinstein, Randi Zinn, Rebecca Soffer, Amy Blumenfeld, Thatcher Wine, Michele Filgate, Eve Rodsky, Beth Ricanti, M.D., Jane Green, Lisa Jewell, Fiona Davis, Julie Satow, Amanda Salzhauer, Holly Peterson, Ingrid Fetell Lee, Camille Pagan, Marisa Bardach Ramel, Claire Bidwell Smith, Jamie Brenner, Sarah McColl, Sen. Kirsten Gillibrand, Helen Ellis, Kathy Wang, Lauren Gershell, Eva Hagberg Fisher, Teresa Sorkin, and Tullan Holmqvist.

I've also moderated the "Women on the Move" series at the Temple Emanu-El Streicker Center, thanks to Marjorie Shuster, with Susan Isaacs, Jennifer Weiner, Rachel Beanland, Capricia Penavic-Marshall, Judith Viorst, Laura Zigman and Taffy Brodesser-Akner. At PEN America, I interviewed Brit Bennett thanks to Suzanne Nossel.

I've even developed friendships with frequent guests from my past salons like Suzy from *Suzy Approved Book Reviews*, Caroline Waxler (epic dinner once with Glynnis MacNicol and Piper Weiss), Rana Binder, Sara Bliss, Lisa Barr, Lynda Loigman, Susie Orman Schnall, Jackie Friedland, Tori O'Connell, Will Schwalbe, Mark Siegel, and author Georgia Clark, who hosted me for a Generation Women event.

I've gotten to know some amazing editors along the way, too, like Sally Kim at Putnam, the fabulous Jenny Jackson at Knopf/ Doubleday, Jennifer Kasius at Running Press (who told me this book would take far too long to come out to be relevant!), and Serena Jones at Henry Holt.

My girlfriends have been a huge help through this whole thing, especially my Yale '98 crew: Ann Jordan (my go-to for life's travails), Abby Schwartz, Andrea Cheng, Danielle Faris Mahfood and Kate Lane, who took a girls trip to LA with me when I was nominated for a Webby Award and spent the whole trip indulging me in all my marketing brainstorming.

Many of the authors I've interviewed have become (or have been) close or old friends, like Liz Astrof, Elisa Strauss, Lauren Braun Costello, Betsy Carter, Sue Shapiro (my former New School writing class teacher), Rebecca Schrag Hershberg, Jill Zarin (who Kyle has known for years), Jeff Norton, Charles Duhigg and Victoria Montgomery Brown (HBS classmates), Elliot Ackerman (Lea's paramour), Lyss Stern (who I wrote for at the *New York Observer*'s *Playground* magazine), Priscilla Gilman (who was the cool older girl in my grade school), Dylan Lauren (who I've known forever from Round Hill), Jennie Wallace, Cristina Alger (my kids' pre-school!), and Jill Kargman (who I grew up with and knew from Yale).

My many other girlfriends and fellow moms from Juad Masters in preschool to Nicole Harris today, you know who you are and I am so grateful for all of you. Especially my Los Angeles girls, Karen Frankel and Alyson Ein. (Dreaming of Cabo.) Isabelle Krishana, thanks for all the tennis and book recommendations. Jessica Harris for that Sette Mezzo lunch when we confessed all and for your professional role modeling. Meagan Ouderkirk, who I met through my old friend Steve Purdy, has been there for me through it all, just like Peter and Erin Friedland, Maggie Chi, Justin and Shirley Steinberg, Nancy and

Marc Badner, Rachel Goulding, Sarah Saint-Amand, Tara Johnson (dog gifts!), Taylor Margis-Noguera, Sarah Irwin, Rachel Young, Stephanie Kearney, Lillie Howard, Carrie Quinn, Gouri Edlich, Mary Vertin, Eva Heyman, Dana Wallach Jones, Felice Axelrod, and so many others.

Other amazing supporters include my original *Seventeen* editor Rory Evans, Nora Krug from the *Washington Post*, JoAn Monaco, Lisa Rappoport, Shirley Chiang, Christine Shim, Ilana Eck, Carolyn Brody and Jesse Bartel from BookHampton, Mary Dell Harrington and Lisa Heffernan from Grown & Flown, Shoshanna Lonstein Gruss, Lauren Gabrielson, Liz Vaccariello from *Real Simple*, Jennifer Steil, Nora McInerny, Evangeline Lilly, Michael Frank, and Lydia Fenet. Thanks to Jeanne Blasberg for the tote I carry all the time, Emily Nemens for the *Paris Review* T-shirt (!), and Christine Anderson for the referrals. Also to Madeleine Henry, Erika Olson, and to Deborah Burns for the URL and company idea. Thanks to Jordan Newman, Lauren Jarvis and Max Cutler at Spotify, and Ali Ehrlich, Lauren Sher and Caterina Andreano at *GMA*. To Taylor Rose Berry for the books and mimosas. To the Friendlys.

Thanks to Jenny Fischbach for designing our New York apartment, especially my library/office, the happiest room ever. And to Brian Ninnis for whenever anything goes wrong there. Thanks to Heather Karaman and Allison Hermann for the sanity checks. To Melanie Goldberger and Hal Orief for making the Pacific Palisades our home away from home. To Stephanie Freilich and team, and Seth and Heather Gordon, for keeping my kids alive.

Thanks to the late, great Stacey Sanders, my college roommate and best friend who we lost on 9/11, showing me, in every way, how to embrace life. And thanks to her mom, Martha, and sister, Laura, for keeping her in my life by staying in touch. Thanks also to Stacey's close friend Abi Ross, who has shown me what resilience looks like. And to Bryan and Amy Koplin: Bryan for years of love and Amy for choosing such a great guy and for our coffee/advice session. Thanks to Didi Hockstader for staying in touch and keeping Avery's memory alive. Avery was one of my best friends in high school who became mentally ill and threw herself in front of subway one tortured day while I was in business school. I think about her all the time.

Thanks to the Group 6 breakfast club, including our late leader, Paige Hardy. I can still hear Paige telling us about her handsome oncologist and how she told him in her Kentucky accent, "Honey, I can't die. I have five kids." I wish her body had cooperated. I kiss the clock daily at 11:11 and think of Paige, the Hardy Party, and all the joy she brought to our lives before ovarian cancer snatched her away. I miss her.

One last goodbye: to Connie Figueroa, my family's housekeeper since I was ten years old, who was pushed in front of an approaching subway by a mentally ill woman who had just been released from Bellevue. Connie grew up with me. She was nineteen years old when she came to the U.S. from the Phillipines and landed, somehow, in our home. She was a true part of our family for thirty-plus years. I still can't believe that's how her life ended, but I am no stranger to trauma.

Thanks to Jovelyn Valle who I found through 99Designs.com for the podcast logos and cover design, McCain Merren for the cover photo, and Nina Vargas for the inspiration and styling of it.

Special thanks again to Carolyn Murnick, Claire Gibson and Elissa Altman for editing all these amazing essays.

Thanks to more of the moms who have been in the trenches with me past and present like Lisa Blau, Danyelle Freeman, Lily Band, Suzanne Harl, May Olatoye, Devra Martinez, Paige Costigan, Elizabeth Fraise, Tami Gaines, Brooke Harlow, Phoebe Polk, Alex Linden, Ferebee Taube, Charlotte Phillips, Sayuri Ganepola, Jocelyn Chu, Perri Brenner, Kate Bullinger, Jennifer James, Gretchen Englander, Lara Metz, Carter Simonds, Brooke Bancroft,

Katie Sawatzky, Khristina McLaughlin, Danielle Anderman, Julie Smigel, Cary Jackson, Susie Anderson, Augusta Moore, Alieda Keevil, Anne Ford, Amy Tarr, Ashley Reid, Mettrie Lari, Charlotte Kaiser Weinberg, Carey Mangriotis, Erica Martini, Nina Patterson, Vanessa Cornell, Ana Villodres, Debra Steigich, Monica Storch, Ashley Rose, Sara Peters, Cory Cary, Kim Straker, Libby Goldring, Dana Tierney, Allison Koslow, Natasha Boucai, Molly McNairy, Chai Vasarhelyi, Fei Wang, Chrissie Panos, Mindy Webster, Elanna Allen, Heather McAuliffe, Kate Seib, Olivia Wassenaar, Victoria Hays, Zoe Tannenbaum, Nancy Badner, Alexandra Robertson, Caroline Gertler, Caroline Portny, Allison Derfner, Donya Bommer, the Epsteins, Jill Wilpon, Robbin Mitchell, Kat Dines, KK Kravis and Jonny Schulhof, author Teru Clavel, author Sara Bliss, Willa Fawer, Gina Marinelli, Nicole Harris, Aurora Sermoneta, Stephanie Borges, Marianna Sabater, Eva Starr (and Chloe!!!), Whitney Topping, Raja Clark, Isabel Tonelli, Elizabeth Williams, Lisa Frelinghuysen, Nancy Park, Pam (and Jon!) Henes, Luleng Chua, and old friends like Kiki Samuels, Daniella Coules, Lauren Frank, Rebecca Raphael, Lizzie/Katie/Claudia, the Jankes, Anna Kovner and Seth Meisel, Naomi Waletzky, Abby Levy, Andrea Dale, Ellie Reitzes, Lauren Royce, Lara Trafelet, the de la Mottes, Claudio and Irene, Amy Sheehan, Craig and Karin Chapman, the Earls, the Thackers, Don Tudor, the Braffs, the Kwiats, Liz Herzberg, Dolly Geary, the Pantzers, the Fines, the Freundlichs, the Landes, Pam Perskie, the Waldrons, the Kojimas, Jon and Liz Kurpis, Abby Baratta, the Brands, the Warnkens, the Satnicks/Joels, the deFlorios, the Murrays, the Nallys, the Jensens, the Ingalls, the Abrahams, the Burches, the Gishes, the McLellans, the Adams/Caputos, the McBrides, the Korpuses, the Jenkins, the Werners, the Yoseloffs, the Bergers, the Altschulers, Alfredo and Cata, Erin and Damien Blumetti, Frank Bua, Tristana and Grier, Robbie Felice, Joey and Jackie, Alexandra Peterson, Alice and Jay, Jemilah Afshar, the Steinbergs, Marilyn Gans, Nancy Lascher, Melissa Crandall, Amanda

Werner, Amanda Weisser, Amy Yamamoto, the Olshans, Ashley Massengale, Avery Sheffield and Dan Rosenthal, Emily Peterson, Fran Stempler, Heather Hoesch, Kalliope Karella, Katie Zorn, Liz Lange, Monica Joshi, Susan Molloy, Willie Watkins, Ken Wolfe, Nina Christopher, Alden Budill, Amy Rabinowitz, the idealab/PayMyBills team, the Foxes, Ingrid Heidrick, John Maggio and Stacey Swiantek, and Dan O'Keefe, Ed Smith, and the Oaks from 223 days, the Fleisses, Natalie Kaplan, Jess Murphy, Allison Bardeen, the Solomons, Doug and Eva Heyman, Elana Nathan and Aliza Pressman, the Goodys/ Brenners, the Nordemans, Andrea Miller, Anna Mallett, Isabelle Aguerre, the Curiels, all of HBS Section B, Corey Lambert, Matt Klauer, Kara Cohen, Cameron Hughes, Jesse Johnston, Brett and Greg Heyman for the birthday wishes. Thanks to Mindy and Jon Gray for buying all those Nene's Treats.

Thanks to Coach Cass, Annika Pergament, Daisy Prince, and Rev. Lydia Sohn. Thanks to Nicole Ross for sneaking me in.

To all the partners, especially Page 1 Books, Book of the Month Club, the Pick Up Line Media, Jumpstart, BINC, Poets & Writers, Chloe's Fruit, and Hamptons Handpoured.

Thanks to all my followers on Instagram whose comments fuel my daily life. Seriously.

Thanks to all the listeners of *Moms Don't Have Time to Read Books*.

Thanks to my new community of *Moms Don't Have Time to Lose Weight* members and podcast listeners.

Thanks to everyone who reached out and said they were thinking about Kyle, Stef, and me after we/they lost Susan and Nene like Liz from White Fences who dropped off baked goods.

Thanks to the amazing authors who blurbed this book including Lena Dunham, Dani Shapiro, J. Courtney Sullivan, Claire Bidwell Smith, Allison Pataki, Deborah Copaken, Laura Zigman, Stephanie Danler, Nora McInerny, Lori Gottlieb, Bess Kalb, and Lily King.

Thanks to my volunteer launch team: Michele Olson, Amy Furash, Leigh Shulman, Jelena Meisel, Shelli Johannes, Ashley Massengale, Katie Cunningham, Lindsay Okamoto, Rebekah Jacobs, Stacey Mosher Gellen, Alexis Rybny, Rina Brahmbhatt, Tiffany Merriman, Kristi Schmitz, Amanda McNutt, Brooke Adams Law, Tara Ohayon, Christine VanDeVelde, Kristine Lassen, Matt Rosanke, Tamara Schweitzer, Jennifer Howard, Allison Nowak, Susan Yablonksky, Erin Robertson, Mary Marraccini, Tate Whitlinger, Rebecca Friedman, Lauren Gabrielson, Tamara Behan, Teresa Sorkin, Samantha Ekert, Karla Andrew, Marybeth Brock, Elana Storch, Elizabeth Weiss, Laurie Cotumaccio, Leslie Ruminski, Francene Katzen, Mary Sheriff, Lisa Godwin, Ann (A.H.) Kim, Barbara Libbin, Francesca Borin, Bill Dameron, Kara McGee, Bonnie Goldberg, Meghan Jarvis, Melanie Goldberger and Rebecca Macatee. (Team still in formation, so thanks to everyone who joined and helped!)

Thanks to everyone I've ever interviewed! I truly enjoyed getting to know you.

Kyle's team at Morning Moon Productions has been invaluable to me: Dan Lotti, Mike Sivilli, Austen Rydell, Ethan Lazar and Jordan Blumetti. Jordan (who is a phenomenal writer in his own right), Kyle, and I had lunch with our dear friends Cristina Alesci and Stephen Diamond the summer before last, and they all helped me brainstorm how to grow my business. I still use those tips. Dan and Mike have provided the intro and outro music through the Moon Brothers and Dangermuffin to all my podcasts and videos. Anna Claire, Dan's wife, gave me life-saving allergy remedies when we inherited Susan's dogs. Billie Lourd, Austen's fiancee, has been a huge help along the way, too. And Kingston, the first baby moon on the team (well, aside from Luna!). Our epic summer lunch with Billie's dad, Bryan Lourd, and Bruce Bozzi (old family connections from the Palm in the Fred Thimm, Carey Meyer days!) has already led to so much great stuff, including my new podcast representation by CAA agents Josh

Lindgren and Yuni Sher, and so many wonderful introductions from Kate Childs and Cait Hoyt, plus advice from Michelle Weiner. Austen, Ethan and Ethan's girlfriend, Sara, created the backdrop for my many Zoom quarantine calls by arranging all the books by color on my new bookshelf. Ethan has already provided me a lot of strategic counsel; he is whip-smart. And all that food Austen and company sent after Susan passed away? I am still working it off.

I started working with Suzanne Williams and Deb Shapiro at Shreve Williams PR recently for my projects but have been emailing with them for years about their other author clients. I always thought that if I could ever sell a book, they'd be who I'd want to work with. They are, I'm sure, already sick of my nonstop emails. When I thought about doing this book, I decided to pitch exclusively to Skyhorse given their fast turnaround time and expertise. (That coffee at Ralph's!) My editor there, Caroline Russomanno, has been fantastic and tolerant of all my pestering so far, and Kathleen Schmidt has been lovely.

Since the quarantine hit, I've gotten to know so many other authors . . . through my podcast, yes, but also from my *Z-IGTV* Instagram Live show, my *KZ Time* show with Kyle, and *Zibby's Virtual Book Club*, authors like Kevin Kwan, Adrienne Brodeur, Maya Lang, Ruthie Lindsey, Uchechi Mba-Uzoukwu, Terri Cheney, Rachel Barenbaum, Jeanine Cummins, Caitlin Moran, Sue Miller, Chris Bohjalian, Phyllis Grant, Alyssa Shelasky, Elyssa Friedland, Jodie Patterson, Adrienne Bankert and Kristy Woodson Harvey.

Thanks to Celia McGee at the Center for Fiction, Jane Rosen, Lisa Leshne, Torrey Maldonado, Heather Cabot, Shelli Johannes, Naomi Firestone, Cynthia Kitay, Daniel Bokun, Deb Copaken, Deborah Tannen, Brad Meltzer, Laura Munson, Brian Platzer, Jeff Gordinier, Lauren Passell, Leigh Newman, Lisa Taddeo, Lynne and Val Constantine, JJ Ramberg, Alan Silberberg, Vashti Harrison, Karah Preiss, Katie Davidson, Joyce Chang, Julie Valerie, Jeanne

McCulloch, Molly Barton, Jennifer Blecher, Jennifer Gray, Esther Wojcicki, Gary Brody, Robin Homanoff, Emily Raiber, Bettina Elias Siegel, Bill Clegg, Alex Aster, Daniella Pierson, Jenn Risko, Rex Ogle, Eve Rodsky, Elizabeth Gerlach, Alisyn Camerota, Abby Sher, Diane Debrovner, Caroline Leavitt, Jenna Blum, Sally Shaywitz, Tara Kinsey, Andy Dodds, Ali Wenzke, Meredith Hoffa, Richie Jackson, Sandra Miller, Meg Resnikoff, Shannon Twomey, Raakhee Michandani, Jamie Lee Curtis, Laura Tremaine, Caroline Leavitt, Sarah Gelman, Sarah Elison, Kathy Bartson, Hollie Fraser, Rosy Kehdi, Jordana Horn, Andy Hunter, Lisa Belkin, Liz Egan, Anna Halkidis, Beth Kneebone, Jessica Silverster, Rebecca Dube, Gretchen Schreiber, Cynthia Kitay, Amy Impelizzeri, the Book of the Month team, Steve Long, Ashley Hayes, Meagan Briggs, and so, so, so many others.

To Alyson and Morgan Ein, Karen and Eli Frankel, Somsara and David Rielly, Lizzie Friedman, Jenny Lee, Dibs Baer, Nicole and Steve Solaka, Amanda and Sam Brown, Tyler and Talia Friedman, Shannon Olivas, Aaron and Kristin Bendikson, Fritz and Jennie McGuire, Trevor and Evelin Nielsen, Victoria Lobis, and Steven Rowley, in L.A.

Thanks to my Zibby's Virtual Book Club regulars Meghan Jarvis, Alysia Reiner, Cheryl Sokoloff, Sherie Silver, Carol Orange, Francene Katzen, and others. Thanks to Melissa Gould, Emmanuel Acho, Rachel Hollis, Jennifer and David Risher, Jean Kwok, Rachel Bloom, Arden Myrin, Jarrett Krosoczka, Paige Peterson, Kara Goldin, Nessa Rapoport, Matt Bocchi, Cameron Douglas, Liz Petrone, Dr. Jill Biden, Elizabeth Lesser, Christie Tate, Elizabeth Berg, Lauren Tarshis, *and so many more.*

I've also been interviewed by others like complete pros Mallory Kasdan, Anne Bogel, Amy Schmidt, Suzanne Falter, Jordana Horn, Lisa Wexler, Heather Hansen, Biz Ellis, Samhita Jayanti, Ana Kertesz, Matt Hall, Sarah Dickinson, Patrick McGinnis, Brooke Adams-Law, Sandy Abrams, Cheryl Butler, Brandy Ferner, Marti Post, and the entire Pick Up Line team.

To Rabbi Gelfand, Rabbi Davidson and Rabbi Ehrlich, thank you for all your help during our time of intense need. To Ben Kirschenbaum for all the support and teaching.

To Sue Fleming and Cat Guerriere for keeping all of us moving and afloat in so many ways. To Shannon Simpson for everything.

Thanks to Ken Davis at Mount Sinai Health System, who made one phone call that changed everything, Gigi from Round Hill for her expert medical advice, and Lizzie Friedman (again), who connected me to a friend at Duke when I needed it (and for her lifetime of friendship). Thanks to dear friends Evette Ferguson, Gigi Stone Woods, and Sayuri Ganepola for summer "camp" support as things unfolded.

Thanks to Tenzin Palmo Patsatsang, my nanny of thirteen plus years, who takes care of me just as much as she does the kids. Thanks also to newbie Dolma Dawa for helping on weekends. (Also see Jamie Mortimer, above.) Thanks to Zompa Gurung for helping us keep our home clean, cared for, and organized. And to Jesus Santos, the original Zoomer. Also thanks to the many former babysitters who have helped me manage having four kids including Adriana Cutler, Catherine Chambers, Kim Taracena, and Chrystal Gray.

Thank you to my sound editors, Steve Ejbick and Ryan MacNeill from Texturessound, to Sara Grambusch from Bold Transcription, to Trina and Kathy, my business accountants. To Sultanna Singh and Paul White for keeping everything in order. To Allison Guerrero for the quotes. To Social Fleur for the social media consulting. To Kristi Faulkner for creating "Brand Zibby." To Maxi, for the vision.

To all the publicists I email with all the time and who send me amazing guests including Ariele Fredman, Ariane Moore, Jessica Roth, Marian Brown, Katie Bassel, Jane Beirn, Megan Rudloff, Megan Fishman, Claire McLaughlin, Amelia Possanza, Jordan Rodman, Heather Mill, Aileen Boyle, Leslie Cohen, Alexander Kelleher-Nagorski, Ann-Marie Nieves, Kathleen Carter, Ashley Hewlett, Nicole

Dewey, Hannah Bishop, Caitlin Mulrooney-Lyski, Heather Drucker, Crystal Patriache, Martha Kiley, Dini von Mueffling, Christopher Smith, Todd Doughty, Gretchen Koss, Kristin Ilardi, Kamrun Nesa, Keely Platte, Jimmy Harvey, Justine Sha, Sonya Cheuse, and Staci Burt.

To Jade Fontenay for letting me change my mind.

To Margaret Anastas for buying my children's books for Penguin Random House's new imprint, Flamingo, and to Karen Dukess for the intro. Looking forward to Princess Charming!!

Of course, thank you to every single author who wrote a piece for *We Found Time* which has now found its way into this anthology. Thanks for handing in the essays on time, turning in the edits, and writing from your hearts during a period of time in the world when most people were too anxious or terrified to open their laptops. Your words will undoubtedly help so many others, as they did me.

Now for my immediate crew.

To my grandmother, Carol Levitan ("Gagy"), age ninety-seven, who has encouraged me to write from the start and even, with her husband "Papa Kal," published my first mini-book when I was nine years old. I called her recently to check in and see what was new and she quipped, "Well, I'm pregnant."

My favorite podcast guest of all has been my dad, Steve Schwarzman. He wrote a bestselling book last year called *What it Takes*. When I went to his office boardroom and interviewed him on my laptop, he looked over at me, amused, as I set everything up. I then interviewed him for a BookHampton event. My kids sat in the front row with my brother and my niece, Lucy, who seems to be the only one among the cousins and my kids to truly inherit my passion for books. But back to my dad. My dad has given me everything in life, particularly the luxury of being able to pursue my passions, like this entire endeavor. I look to his approval for almost everything I accomplish. After all, I don't want him to think I'm "sitting around eating bonbons." His nonstop work ethic infuses everything I do. My zest-for-life stepmother Christine was a huge help when Susan was in the hospital and always, and my stepsister Megan helped so much with the dogs.

My mom, Ellen Katz, has been a truly enormous lifelong support, and was the one who originally made me submit my first essay to *Seventeen* magazine. I forgive her now for snooping into what I was writing. I also credit her with fostering my love of reading, taking me to the East Hampton Library over and over again, refilling that L.L.Bean tote bag. She attends many of my events now, online and in-person, even though I don't always call on her when she raises her hand. Her unwavering support and Midwestern values have kept me centered my whole life. Howard, my amazing stepdad who I love so much, and his kids Betsey Katz (and the fabulous Amanda Brand!), and Sara (and Doug) Mercer have been really great. I often think about Adam, who we lost far too young, and try to feed Zach Katz whenever he'll let me. Who knew I'd have a step-nephew who towers over me?! My aunts, uncles and cousins have been a delightfully wonderful support. When they tell me they're proud of me, it really means something to me. I hope they know that: Aunt Nancie and Uncle Mark, Uncle Tom and Aunty Marty, Uncle Warren and Aunt Ginny, Zak and Christi, Alexandra (and Mike), Caroline, Ashley, Carrie, Spencer and Julia, and Luisa Kingsdale.

My "little" brother, Teddy Schwarzman, crushed me professionally for so long with his amazing production company, Black Bear Pictures. Watching his film *The Imitation Game* win an Academy Award and spotting Teds and his wife, Ellen, at the ceremony on TV was a life highlight for me. Last summer, they whisked Kyle, the kids, and me to Montana as Susan was in dire straits, a birthday surprise. I'll never forget their generosity and love when we needed it the most. Teds, I was so blessed to have grown up with you ("Hefty, Hefty, Cinch-Sack!") and am even more blessed to be growing older with you. Ellen, Lucy ("kid!"), William, and Mary, I love you all.

To Stefanie, my sister-in-law, for braving this journey together—and for all the dog treats. I'm so glad we wear the same shoe size. And I'm beyond happy you stayed in New York. To Bernard and Miriam, let's keep laughing together.

To my ex, Andrew, for bringing the kids into the world—and for taking them every other weekend.

To my ex-sister-in-law but forever sister, I love you, Elizabeth.

To Kyle, for literally everything. The idea. The encouragement. The laughs. The advice. The creativity. The collaboration. (I can't wait for the books you've optioned from the podcast to come to life!) The love. The *Shark Tank* episodes. The Advil late at night. The coffee. The emojis during Instagram Lives. The hugs. The stepfathering. The meals!!!!!! You've fed my body and soul in every way since the day I met you. I am me because of you. You are it.

And to my kids: O, P, S, and G. I know you don't always like it that I do so many podcasts when I could be hanging out with you in the next room, and that you often tell me to put down the book I'm reading so I can play with you. I hope the fact that I interview so many of your favorite authors, too, helps! I hope you'll remember all the good I'm trying to bring into the world. I hope you'll find something you're equally passionate about when you grow up. I hope you'll work as hard as I do and give back even more. And, above all, I hope you know that nothing is more important than you. When you say you're proud of me, which you all have at different times and in different ways, it "fills my bucket." I love you, truly, more than words can say. And no, one of you is *not* my favorite. You are the most special group of four people on this planet. I can't wait to stand by and see what you all do with your amazing talents and beautiful souls. You are everything. Full stop. (Wait, is today a Wednesday frap day?!)

Thanks, everyone. Thank you, thank you, thank you. I know, even though I've gone through my inboxes and memory bank, I've forgotten key people. If you're one of them, I'm so sorry. I appreciate it. And I especially appreciate every single person who has read this book. Thank you for spending time with all of us.

One final thank-you to all the authors not mentioned who have ever written a book I've read that has delighted, entertained, challenged, taught, helped, tickled, or transported me. I am eternally grateful.

See? Aren't you glad you found time to read the acknowledgments?

Xx,
Zibby

ABOUT THE EDITOR

Zibby Owens is the creator and host of award-winning podcast *Moms Don't Have Time to Read Books.* Zibby, named "NYC's Most Powerful Book-fluencer" by *Vulture,* conducts warm, inquisitive conversations with authors. Before the pandemic, Zibby ran a literary salon, hosted her own book fairs, and was a frequent bookstore event moderator.

During the quarantine, Zibby hosted two Instagram Live author talk shows, launched an online magazine with original author-written essays called *We Found Time,* and started Zibby's Virtual Book Club.

Zibby has recommended books for the *Washington Post, Good Morning America,* and *Real Simple.* She has also contributed to *Parents, Marie Claire, Redbook,* the *New York Times* online, and many other publications.

Zibby has appeared on *CBS This Morning, Good Morning America,* the BBC, ABC-7 *Eyewitness News, Good Day LA, Good Day DC, Good Day Dallas,* and other local news outlets.

She has two children's books coming out in 2022, plus a second anthology coming out in November 2021 called *Moms Also Don't Have Time To.*

Zibby recently launched an Instagram community and podcast called *Moms Don't Have Time to Lose Weight.*

Zibby serves on the board of trustees at the Child Mind Institute, the Mount Sinai Health System, and the Mount Sinai Parenting

Center, and cochairs the Library Council of the New York Public Library.

A graduate of Yale University and Harvard Business School, Zibby currently lives in New York with her husband, Kyle Owens of Morning Moon Productions, and her four children, ages six to thirteen. She always has a book nearby.

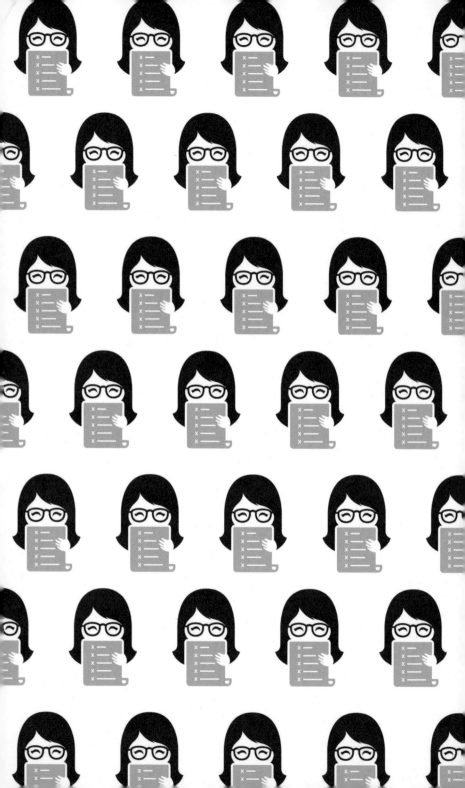